Anatomy and Physiology Applied to Obstetrics

For Churchill Livingstone:

Publisher: Mary Law
Copy Editor: Sukie Hunter
Production Controller: Nancy Henry
Sales Promotion Executive: Hilary Brown

Anatomy and Physiology Applied to Obstetrics

Sylvia Verralls SRN SCM MTD

Formerly: Principal Midwifery Tutor, North Middlesex Hospital;
Assistant Training Officer, N.E. Met. Regional Health Authority;
Lecturer, Health and Social Service Studies, Worthing College
of Technology, Worthing

THIRD EDITION

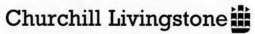

Churchill Livingstone

EDINBURGH LONDON MADRID MELBOURNE NEW YORK AND
TOKYO 1993

CHURCHILL LIVINGSTONE
Medical Division of Longman Group UK Limited

Distributed in the United States of America by Churchill Livingstone Inc.,
650 Avenue of the Americas, New York, N.Y. 10011, and by associated
companies, branches and representatives throughout the world.

First edition 1969 (Pitman Publishing Ltd)
Second edition 1980 (Pitman Publishing Ltd)
Third edition 1993
  Reprinted 1994

ISBN   0-443-04211-X

British Library Cataloguing in Publication Data
A catalogue record for this book is available from the British Library.

Library of Congress Cataloging in Publication Data
A catalog record for this book is available from the Library of Congress.

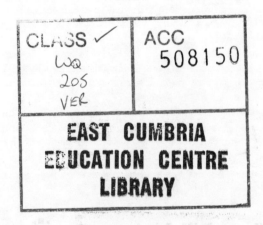

The
publisher's
policy is to use
**paper manufactured
from sustainable forests**

Produced by Longman Singapore Publishers Pte. Ltd.
Printed in Singapore

Preface

A great many people have contributed to the publication of this long overdue third edition and without their aid my task would have been quite impossible.

First I must thank the many midwife teachers and the representatives from allied professions who responded to our requests regarding the subject matter and presentation of the new edition. To meet their wishes, the simple form of presentation and line diagrams have been retained as far as possible, whilst updating of the text has been carried out and some topics have been covered in greater depth to suit current requirements. The primary objective of the text remains unchanged, namely, to teach anatomical facts and relate them to the practical work of the midwife. To comply with the wishes of those tutors who asked for at least one better detailed illustration to supplement each chapter some works of F. Netter have been included in a Plate section and I am grateful to the Ciba Foundation for allowing us to reproduce them.

To Miss Averil Mitchell, the tutors and staff, including the librarians, of Southlands Hospital, Shoreham-by-Sea I owe a great deal of gratitude. Miss Mitchell gave unstintingly of her time and there must have been occasions when the staff thought I had become part of the furniture.

Similar thanks must be extended to Sister Christine NSSJD and the teaching staff of Greenwich District Hospital. The painstaking reading of draft manuscripts together with constructive criticism must inevitably have occupied a great deal of time. I really have appreciated enormously the assistance of both midwifery schools. At a later stage, Miss Sinead McNally, Tutor, Lothian College of Nursing and Midwifery, made valuable comments on the text.

To Mary Emmerson Law and Graham Birnie of Churchill Livingstone, who have borne with my moods of depression, frustration and ill temper when nothing seemed to go right, I extend my sincere apologies as well as my grateful thanks.

It comes with my best wishes to the next generation of student midwives as they learn to practise the art of 'being with the woman' in this last decade of the century.

Ferring 1993   S.V.

Acknowledgements

We are grateful to the CIBA Pharmaceutical Company for permission to reproduce the plates from Netter F H *The CIBA Collection of Medical Illustrations, Volume 2 – Reproductive System*.

We also acknowledge the permission of Sir John Dewhurst and Dr G. Chamberlain to reproduce illustrations from *A Practice of Obstetrics and Gynaecology* (Pitman Publishing Ltd and Churchill Livingstone).

Thanks are also due to V. Ruth Bennett and Linda K. Brown for permission to reproduce illustrations from *Myles Textbook for Midwives* 11th edn (Churchill Livingstone).

Contents

Contents

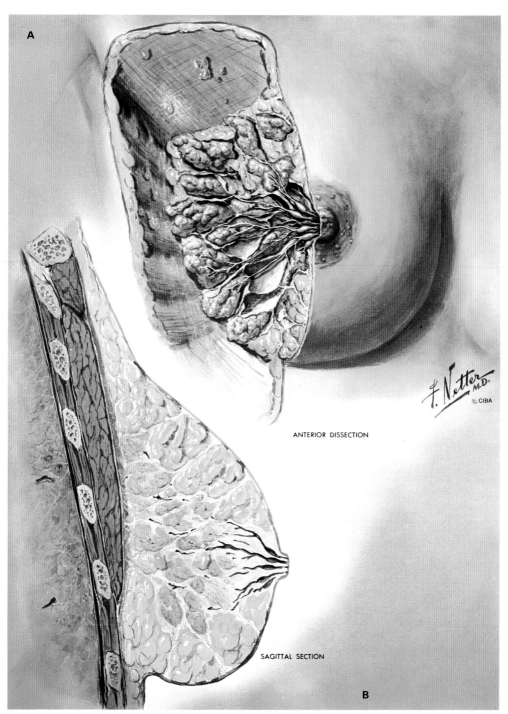

A

ANTERIOR DISSECTION

SAGITTAL SECTION

B

Plate 1 Position and structure of the breast.
(© 1965 CIBA-GEIGY Corporation. Reprinted with permission from The CIBA Collection of Medical Illustrations, illustrated by Frank H. Netter, MD. All rights reserved.)

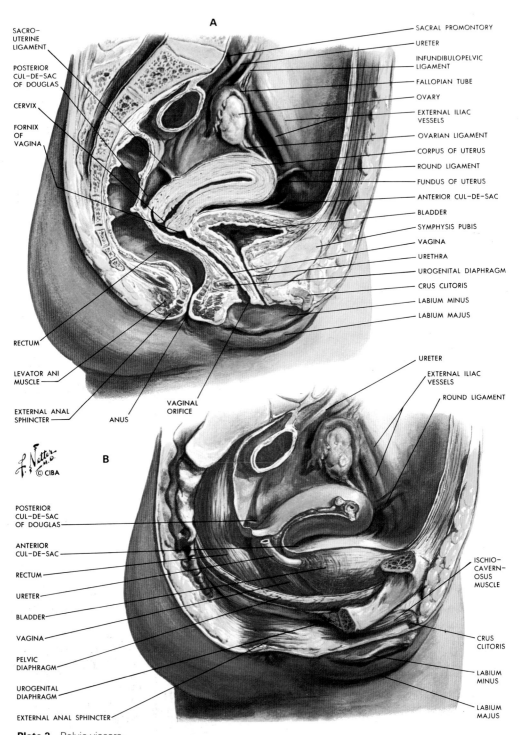

A

SACRO-
UTERINE
LIGAMENT

POSTERIOR
CUL-DE-SAC
OF DOUGLAS

CERVIX

FORNIX
OF
VAGINA

RECTUM

LEVATOR ANI
MUSCLE

EXTERNAL ANAL
SPHINCTER

ANUS

VAGINAL
ORIFICE

SACRAL PROMONTORY

URETER

INFUNDIBULOPELVIC
LIGAMENT

FALLOPIAN TUBE

OVARY

EXTERNAL ILIAC
VESSELS

OVARIAN LIGAMENT

CORPUS OF UTERUS

ROUND LIGAMENT

FUNDUS OF UTERUS

ANTERIOR CUL-DE-SAC

BLADDER

SYMPHYSIS PUBIS

VAGINA

URETHRA

UROGENITAL DIAPHRAGM

CRUS CLITORIS

LABIUM MINUS

LABIUM MAJUS

URETER

EXTERNAL ILIAC
VESSELS

ROUND LIGAMENT

B

POSTERIOR
CUL-DE-SAC
OF DOUGLAS

ANTERIOR
CUL-DE-SAC

RECTUM

URETER

BLADDER

VAGINA

PELVIC
DIAPHRAGM

UROGENITAL
DIAPHRAGM

EXTERNAL ANAL SPHINCTER

ISCHIO-
CAVERN-
OSUS
MUSCLE

CRUS
CLITORIS

LABIUM
MINUS

LABIUM
MAJUS

Plate 2   Pelvic viscera.
(© 1965 CIBA-GEIGY Corporation. Reprinted with permission from The CIBA Collection of Medical
Illustrations, illustrated by Frank H. Netter, MD. All rights reserved.)

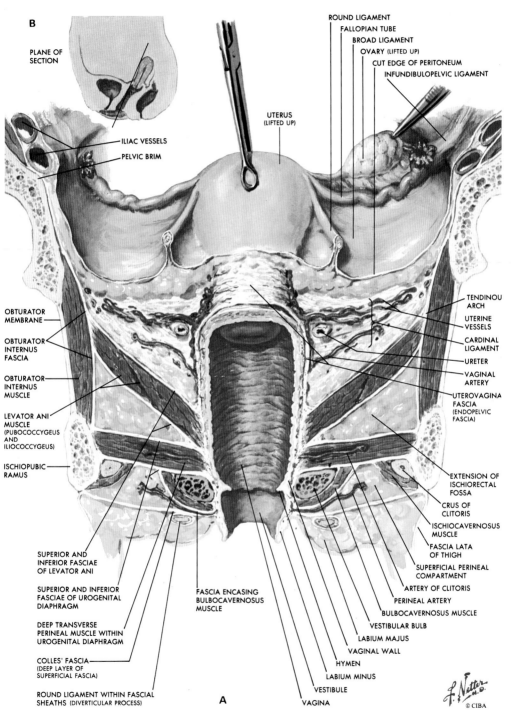

B

PLANE OF SECTION

ROUND LIGAMENT
FALLOPIAN TUBE
BROAD LIGAMENT
OVARY (LIFTED UP)
CUT EDGE OF PERITONEUM
INFUNDIBULOPELVIC LIGAMENT

ILIAC VESSELS
PELVIC BRIM

UTERUS (LIFTED UP)

OBTURATOR MEMBRANE

OBTURATOR INTERNUS FASCIA

OBTURATOR INTERNUS MUSCLE

LEVATOR ANI MUSCLE (PUBOCOCCYGEUS AND ILIOCOCCYGEUS)

ISCHIOPUBIC RAMUS

TENDINOU ARCH
UTERINE VESSELS
CARDINAL LIGAMENT
URETER
VAGINAL ARTERY
UTEROVAGINA FASCIA (ENDOPELVIC FASCIA)

EXTENSION OF ISCHIORECTAL FOSSA
CRUS OF CLITORIS
ISCHIOCAVERNOSUS MUSCLE
FASCIA LATA OF THIGH
SUPERFICIAL PERINEAL COMPARTMENT
ARTERY OF CLITORIS
PERINEAL ARTERY
BULBOCAVERNOSUS MUSCLE
VESTIBULAR BULB
LABIUM MAJUS
VAGINAL WALL
HYMEN
LABIUM MINUS
VESTIBULE
VAGINA

SUPERIOR AND INFERIOR FASCIAE OF LEVATOR ANI

SUPERIOR AND INFERIOR FASCIAE OF UROGENITAL DIAPHRAGM

DEEP TRANSVERSE PERINEAL MUSCLE WITHIN UROGENITAL DIAPHRAGM

COLLES' FASCIA (DEEP LAYER OF SUPERFICIAL FASCIA)

ROUND LIGAMENT WITHIN FASCIAL SHEATHS (DIVERTICULAR PROCESS)

FASCIA ENCASING BULBOCAVERNOSUS MUSCLE

A

f. Netter M.D.
© CIBA

Plate 3 Ligamentous and fascial support of pelvic viscera.

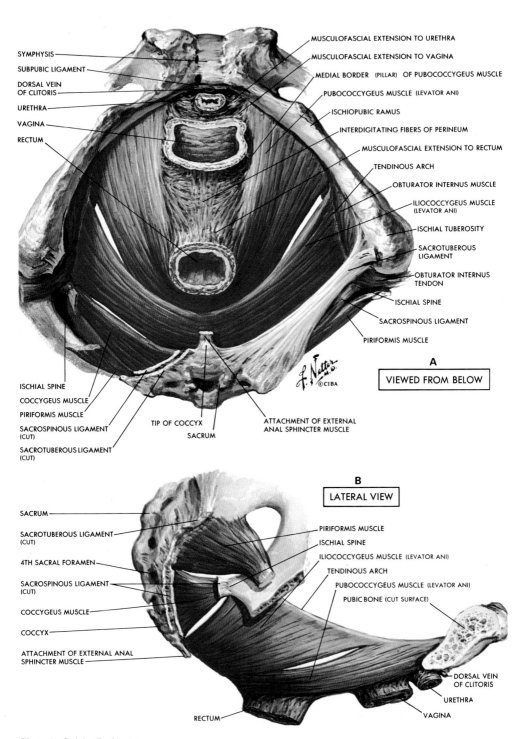

SYMPHYSIS

SUBPUBIC LIGAMENT

DORSAL VEIN OF CLITORIS

URETHRA

VAGINA

RECTUM

MUSCULOFASCIAL EXTENSION TO URETHRA

MUSCULOFASCIAL EXTENSION TO VAGINA

MEDIAL BORDER (PILLAR) OF PUBOCOCCYGEUS MUSCLE

PUBOCOCCYGEUS MUSCLE (LEVATOR ANI)

ISCHIOPUBIC RAMUS

INTERDIGITATING FIBERS OF PERINEUM

MUSCULOFASCIAL EXTENSION TO RECTUM

TENDINOUS ARCH

OBTURATOR INTERNUS MUSCLE

ILIOCOCCYGEUS MUSCLE (LEVATOR ANI)

ISCHIAL TUBEROSITY

SACROTUBEROUS LIGAMENT

OBTURATOR INTERNUS TENDON

ISCHIAL SPINE

SACROSPINOUS LIGAMENT

PIRIFORMIS MUSCLE

A

VIEWED FROM BELOW

ISCHIAL SPINE

COCCYGEUS MUSCLE

PIRIFORMIS MUSCLE

SACROSPINOUS LIGAMENT (CUT)

SACROTUBEROUS LIGAMENT (CUT)

TIP OF COCCYX

SACRUM

ATTACHMENT OF EXTERNAL ANAL SPHINCTER MUSCLE

B

LATERAL VIEW

SACRUM

SACROTUBEROUS LIGAMENT (CUT)

4TH SACRAL FORAMEN

SACROSPINOUS LIGAMENT (CUT)

COCCYGEUS MUSCLE

COCCYX

ATTACHMENT OF EXTERNAL ANAL SPHINCTER MUSCLE

PIRIFORMIS MUSCLE

ISCHIAL SPINE

ILIOCOCCYGEUS MUSCLE (LEVATOR ANI)

TENDINOUS ARCH

PUBOCOCCYGEUS MUSCLE (LEVATOR ANI)

PUBIC BONE (CUT SURFACE)

DORSAL VEIN OF CLITORIS

URETHRA

VAGINA

RECTUM

Plate 4 Pelvic diaphragm.

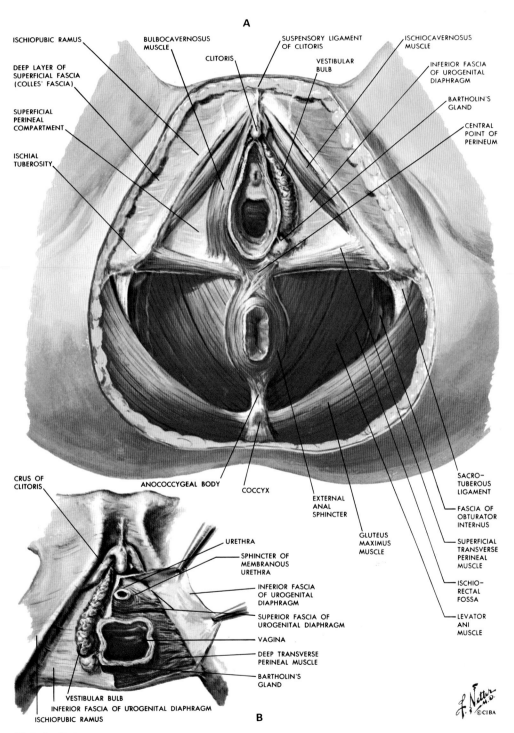

A

ISCHIOPUBIC RAMUS

DEEP LAYER OF
SUPERFICIAL FASCIA
(COLLES' FASCIA)

SUPERFICIAL
PERINEAL
COMPARTMENT

ISCHIAL
TUBEROSITY

BULBOCAVERNOSUS
MUSCLE

CLITORIS

SUSPENSORY LIGAMENT
OF CLITORIS

VESTIBULAR
BULB

ISCHIOCAVERNOSUS
MUSCLE

INFERIOR FASCIA
OF UROGENITAL
DIAPHRAGM

BARTHOLIN'S
GLAND

CENTRAL
POINT OF
PERINEUM

CRUS OF
CLITORIS

ANOCOCCYGEAL BODY

COCCYX

EXTERNAL
ANAL
SPHINCTER

GLUTEUS
MAXIMUS
MUSCLE

SACRO-
TUBEROUS
LIGAMENT

FASCIA OF
OBTURATOR
INTERNUS

SUPERFICIAL
TRANSVERSE
PERINEAL
MUSCLE

ISCHIO-
RECTAL
FOSSA

LEVATOR
ANI
MUSCLE

URETHRA

SPHINCTER OF
MEMBRANOUS
URETHRA

INFERIOR FASCIA
OF UROGENITAL
DIAPHRAGM

SUPERIOR FASCIA OF
UROGENITAL DIAPHRAGM

VAGINA

DEEP TRANSVERSE
PERINEAL MUSCLE

BARTHOLIN'S
GLAND

VESTIBULAR BULB

INFERIOR FASCIA OF UROGENITAL DIAPHRAGM

ISCHIOPUBIC RAMUS

B

F. Netter
M.D.
©CIBA

Plate 5 Perineum.
(© 1965 CIBA-GEIGY Corporation. Reprinted with permission from The CIBA Collection of Medical
Illustrations, illustrated by Frank H. Netter, MD. All rights reserved.)

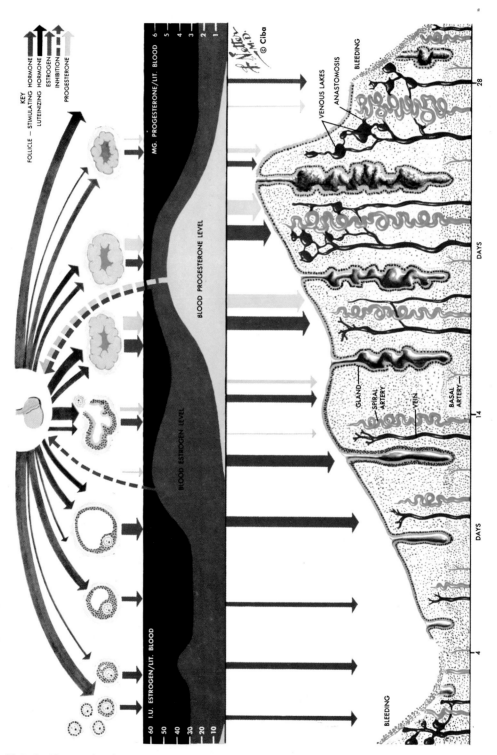

Plate 6 Menstrual cycle.
(© 1965 CIBA-GEIGY Corporation. Reprinted with permission from The CIBA Collection of Medical Illustrations, illustrated by Frank H. Netter, MD. All rights reserved.)

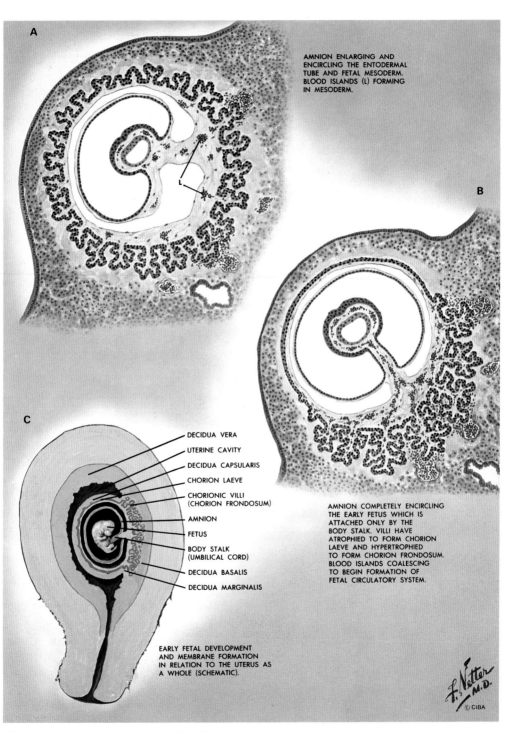

AMNION ENLARGING AND ENCIRCLING THE ENTODERMAL TUBE AND FETAL MESODERM. BLOOD ISLANDS (L) FORMING IN MESODERM.

AMNION COMPLETELY ENCIRCLING THE EARLY FETUS WHICH IS ATTACHED ONLY BY THE BODY STALK. VILLI HAVE ATROPHIED TO FORM CHORION LAEVE AND HYPERTROPHIED TO FORM CHORION FRONDOSUM. BLOOD ISLANDS COALESCING TO BEGIN FORMATION OF FETAL CIRCULATORY SYSTEM.

DECIDUA VERA
UTERINE CAVITY
DECIDUA CAPSULARIS
CHORION LAEVE
CHORIONIC VILLI (CHORION FRONDOSUM)
AMNION
FETUS
BODY STALK (UMBILICAL CORD)
DECIDUA BASALIS
DECIDUA MARGINALIS

EARLY FETAL DEVELOPMENT AND MEMBRANE FORMATION IN RELATION TO THE UTERUS AS A WHOLE (SCHEMATIC).

Plate 7   Development of placenta and fetal membrane.

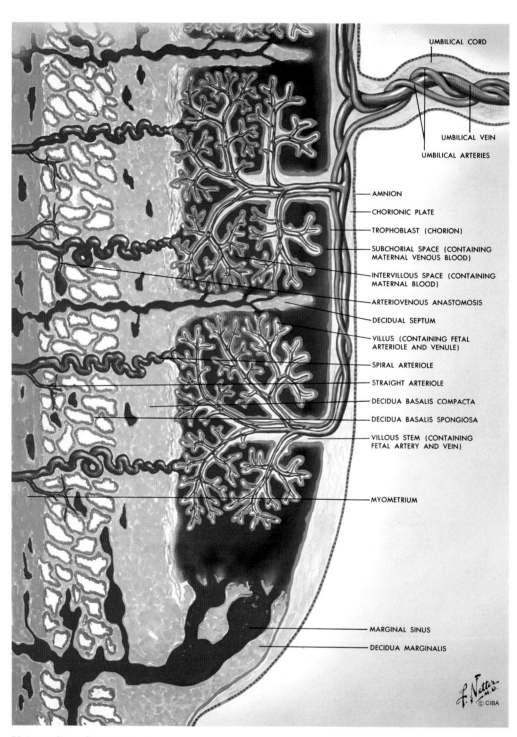

UMBILICAL CORD

UMBILICAL VEIN

UMBILICAL ARTERIES

AMNION

CHORIONIC PLATE

TROPHOBLAST (CHORION)

SUBCHORIAL SPACE (CONTAINING MATERNAL VENOUS BLOOD)

INTERVILLOUS SPACE (CONTAINING MATERNAL BLOOD)

ARTERIOVENOUS ANASTOMOSIS

DECIDUAL SEPTUM

VILLUS (CONTAINING FETAL ARTERIOLE AND VENULE)

SPIRAL ARTERIOLE

STRAIGHT ARTERIOLE

DECIDUA BASALIS COMPACTA

DECIDUA BASALIS SPONGIOSA

VILLOUS STEM (CONTAINING FETAL ARTERY AND VEIN)

MYOMETRIUM

MARGINAL SINUS

DECIDUA MARGINALIS

Plate 8 Circulation in placenta.

1 The female breasts

(Plates 1A and B)

The female breasts, also known as the mammary glands, are accessory organs of reproduction.

Situation One breast is situated on each side of the sternum and extends between the levels of the second and sixth rib. The breasts lie in the superficial fascia of the chest wall over the pectoralis major muscle, and are stabilised by suspensory ligaments.

Shape Each breast is a hemispherical swelling and has a tail of tissue extending towards the axilla (**the axillary tail of Spence**).

Size The size varies with each individual and with the stage of development as well as with age. It is not uncommon for one breast to be a little larger than the other.

Gross structure
(Fig. 1.1)

The axillary tail is the breast tissue extending towards the axilla.

The areola is a circular area of loose, pigmented skin about 2.5 cm in diameter

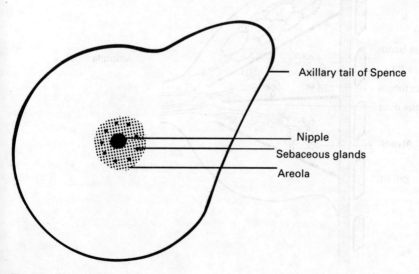

Axillary tail of Spence

Nipple
Sebaceous glands
Areola

Fig. 1.1 Gross structure of the breast.

at the centre of each breast. It is a pale pink colour in a fair-skinned woman, darker in a brunette, the colour deepening with pregnancy. Within the area of the areola lie approximately 20 sebaceous glands. In pregnancy these enlarge and are known as **Montgomery's tubercles**.

The nipple lies in the centre of the areola at the level of the fourth rib. A protuberance about 6 mm in length, composed of pigmented erectile tissue, it is a highly sensitive structure. The surface of the nipple is perforated by small orifices, the openings of the lactiferous ducts. It is covered with epithelium.

Microscopic structure
(Plate 1 & Fig. 1.2)

The breast is composed largely of glandular tissue, but also of some fatty tissue, and is covered with skin. This glandular tissue is divided into about 18 lobes which are completely separated by bands of fibrous tissue. The internal structure is said to resemble the segments of a halved grapefruit or orange. Each lobe is a self-contained working unit and is composed of the following structures.

Alveoli: containing the milk-secreting cells. Each alveolus is lined by milk-secreting cells, the **acini**, which extract from the mammary blood supply the factors essential for milk formation (see Production of Milk, p. 8). Around each alveolus lie myoepithelial cells,

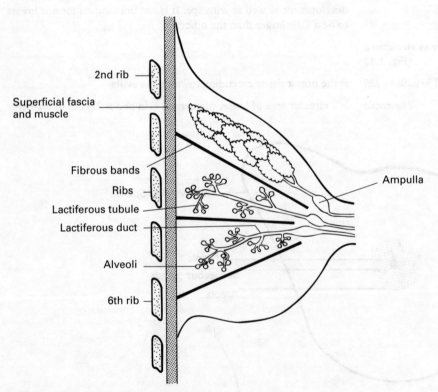

Fig. 1.2 Microscopic structure of the breast.

2nd rib

Superficial fascia and muscle

Fibrous bands

Ribs

Lactiferous tubule

Lactiferous duct

Alveoli

6th rib

Ampulla

sometimes called 'basket' or 'spider' cells. When these cells are stimulated by oxytocin they contract, releasing milk into the lactiferous duct.

Lactiferous tubules: small ducts which connect the alveoli.

Lactiferous duct: a central duct into which the tubules run.

Ampulla: the widened-out portion of the duct where milk is stored. The ampullae lie under the areola.

Continuation of each lactiferous duct: extending from the ampulla and opening on to the nipple.

Blood supply Blood is supplied to the breast by the **internal mammary artery**, the **external mammary artery** and the upper intercostal arteries. Venous drainage is through corresponding vessels into the **internal mammary** and **axillary veins**.

Lymphatic drainage This is largely into the **axillary glands**, with some drainage into the portal fissure of the liver and mediastinal glands. The lymphatic vessels of each breast communicate with one another.

Nerve supply The function of the breast is largely controlled by hormone activity but the skin is supplied by branches of the thoracic nerves. There is also some sympathetic nerve supply, especially around the areola and nipple.

STAGES OF BREAST DEVELOPMENT (Fig. 1.3)

Intrauterine life Primary breast development occurs in both sexes and commences at about the 4th week of intrauterine life. A longitudinal ridge of thickened ectoderm appears on the ventral wall of the fetus, extending between the arm and limb buds on each side. This is the **mammary** or **milk ridge**. Normally it is only in the thoracic region that there is continued development of this ridge; the rest of the cells undergo degeneration. About 2 weeks later, there is some intrusion of the ridge cells in the thoracic region into the underlying mesoderm. Some 20 **mammary buds** are thus developed. Towards the end of pregnancy the buds canalise to form the primitive milk-secreting cells (**alveoli** and **acini**), **lactiferous ducts** and **myoepithelial cells**.

A depressed area known as the **mammary pit** forms where the lactiferous ducts open; the cells here will form the **nipple**. The nipple is sometimes depressed at birth, particularly in pre-term infants, but will become everted when the underlying mesoderm develops. Failure of the mammary pit to surface soon after birth results in an inverted nipple (see p. 15). The **areola** appears as proliferation of the mesoderm occurs towards full term.

Occasionally, some cells of the mammary ridge fail to degenerate and consequently extra breasts or nipples may develop along the

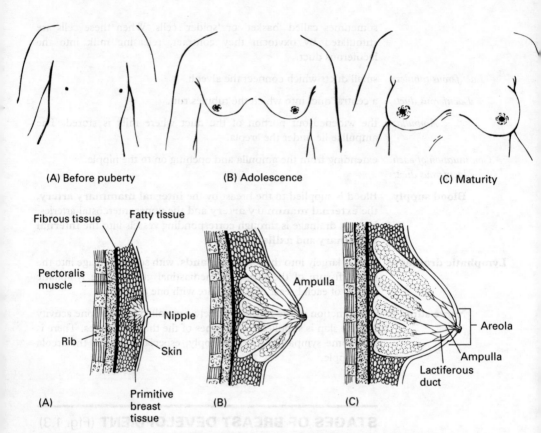

Fig. 1.3   Stages of breast development: (A) Before puberty (B) Adolescence (C) Maturity.

line of the mammary ridge. Extra breasts may not become obvious until pregnancy changes occur. Extra nipples with no surrounding breast tissue may be mistaken for moles.

At birth   Because of the action of maternal hormones circulating in the infant's bloodstream, the breast tissue sometimes is enlarged during the first few days of life. This is due to the withdrawal of maternal hormones from the infant's blood stream. The condition (**mastosis**) may arise in male as well as female infants and is accompanied by milk secretion ('witches' milk). Anxious parents should be reassured that this is only a temporary phenomenon and given an explanation. The condition requires no treatment, for the swelling will subside and milk secretion will ceases as maternal hormones are withdrawn and the infant's own hormone level becomes adjusted.

Following the neonatal period there is normally no activity of breast tissue until puberty (Fig. 1.3A).

At puberty (Fig. 1.3B)   With the rise of hormone levels in females at puberty further development of the breasts occurs and usually precedes the onset of menstruation by about 2 years. Rising oestrogen levels stimulate growth of the lactiferous vessels and the nipple and areola become more pronounced. Rising amounts of progesterone stimulate proliferation of the alveoli. The amounts of fat and fibrous tissue are increased, fat accounting largely for the increase in breast size.

Childbearing years
(Fig. 1.3C)

In the latter half of the menstrual cycle many women, during their childbearing years, complain of breast changes similar to those taking place in pregnancy. These changes are caused by the progesterone produced by the corpus luteum, and soon disappear with the onset of the menstrual flow and decreasing progesterone levels.

Pregnancy

Breast changes are one of the earliest signs of pregnancy and occur in response first to oestrogen, then to progesterone from the corpus luteum and then to hormones from the developing placenta. Stimulus by pregnancy oestrogens results in further development of the nipple and areola and growth of the lactiferous tubules and ducts. In non-pregnant, non-lactating women, the alveoli are small and solid, being filled with granular tissue. In pregnancy, progesterone first causes proliferation of the alveoli in preparation for milk production and then their enlargement and further multiplication.

6th to 8th weeks of pregnancy

The soft tissues of the breast become more nodular to the touch. There is a sensation of fullness, tenderness and tingling – many women dislike their breasts being touched at this period of pregnancy. As the blood supply is increased, the subcutaneous veins become more clearly visible.

12 weeks

Pigmentation of the nipple and areola becomes darker and both become more accentuated. The sebaceous glands lying within the areola enlarge and secrete sebum, an oily substance which lubricates the nipple. At this stage the glands are known as **Montgomery's tubercles. Colostrum** may start to leak from the nipples of a multigravid patient who has successfully breast fed previously. The primigravida will not produce colostrum until later in pregnancy. Its function at this stage, as the precursor of milk, is to prepare the secreting structures and lactiferous vessels for a free flow of milk postnatally. At first it appears as a clear watery fluid.

After 16 weeks

A mottled area surrounding the areola appears and is known as the **secondary areola**. It is more pronounced in dark-haired women. Following childbirth it disappears. True colostrum appears after the 16th week. It becomes more yellow in colour and has a more creamy consistency. The granular tissue in the centre of the alveoli, having undergone fatty degeneration, is now being eliminated as colostrum corpuscles.

Postnatal period

It is only when lactation has been established and is being maintained that the mammary glands can be regarded as fully functioning organs.

COLOSTRUM

It has already been noted:

1. That colostrum is secreted during pregnancy and appears earlier in those mothers whose breasts have already been fully functional.
2. When first produced it is as a clear watery fluid, but it becomes more yellow in appearance and more like thin cream in consistency towards the end of pregnancy.

Following delivery of the infant, its appearance continues to change until by the 3rd postnatal day it looks more like milk, paler in colour and thinner in consistency. This is a transitional phase, for the progression to true milk may take some 10–14 days.

Composition   An average daily sample of colostrum will contain:

Protein 8.5%	Mineral salts 0.4%
Fat 2.5%	Water 85.1%
Carbohydrate 3.5%	Leucocytes
Colostrum corpuscles	Dead epithelial casts

Vitamins A, B, C, D, E and very low levels of vitamin K
Calorific value = 84 kilojoules per 30 ml.

There will of course be variations in these proportions, not only among individual women, but also in the same woman at different times of the day and even during one feed.

Allowing the infant to suckle whenever he appears hungry (**demand feeding**) and for as long as he desires will not only satisfy him but will stimulate production of prolactin and hasten the production of true milk, increase its quantity and help to establish the neurohormonal (milk-ejection or let-down) reflex (Howie & McNeilly 1980).

Functions   As well as preparing the secretory system of the breast for the production of milk, early feeds of colostrum help to clear the infant's intestines of meconium. It is also nutritive and protective.

Nutrition   Colostrum has a high proportion of protein, is highly nutritious and provides all that the infant needs in his early days of life. He should be put to the breast as soon as possible after delivery and then whenever he shows signs of hunger. The length of time at the breast should be unrestricted and the first breast should be emptied before he is put to the other. No complementary or supplementary feeds of cow's milk or water are necessary in most cases.

Protection   Although the infant receives, through the placenta, protection from the diseases to which his mother is immune, antibodies to *E. coli* do not pass through the placental barrier and he is therefore susceptible to diseases such as gastroenteritis.

Colostrum, nevertheless, contains many factors which help to prevent neonatal infections.

Immunoglobulins

The protein fraction of colostrum contains antibodies similar to those which the mother has in her own blood and which protect the infant against bacterial and viral illnesses from which the mother herself has suffered or to which she has an immunity. They act locally in the intestinal tract and can also be absorbed through the intestinal walls into the infant's circulatory system. They also line the intestine and so prevent the absorption of proteins which might cause allergic reactions.

Lactoferrin

This is a protein with a high affinity for iron. Together with one of immunoglobulins (Ig A), lactoferrin takes up the iron which *E. coli*, staphylococci and the yeasts require to flourish. The highest concentration of lactoferrin in colostrum and breast milk is in the first 7 postpartum days. The low iron content of colostrum and breast milk also hinders development of pathogens.

Lactoferrin is present in cow's milk but is destroyed in the pasteurisation process. It is not present in formula feeds.

The immunological effect of lactoferrin would be nullified if the infant's feeds were to be supplemented with iron.

Lysosome

This, together with Ig A, has a non-specific antibacterial function and also inhibits the growth of many viruses. Its concentration in colostrum and breast milk far exceeds that in cow's milk.

Antitrypsin factor

The enzyme **trypsin** is present in the intestinal tract where its function is to break down proteins. The presence of the antitrypsin factor in colostrum and breast milk inhibits the action of trypsin and ensures that protective immunoglobulins are not destroyed.

Bifidus factor

Lactobacilli are present in the infant's intestines and these produce acids which prevent the growth of pathogenic organisms such as the *E. coli* dysentery bacillus, and yeasts such as *Candida albicans* which cause thrush.

In order to flourish, lactobacilli require a nitrogen-containing sugar, the bifidus factor. This factor is present in colostrum and breast milk. It is not present in cow's milk. It is therefore important that the infant's first feeds are of colostrum since lactobacilli are inhibited by cow's milk. Even one feed of cow's milk can affect the intestinal flora detrimentally for as long as 3 days.

These protective factors are all present in mature milk as well as in colostrum. Their concentration alters during the period of lactation as the infant begins to develop his own immunological system. It is worth repeating here:

1. *Early feeds of colostrum* and a continuous supply of breast milk

for at least 4 months are the best protection against disease that the newborn infant can be given

2. *Even just one feed of cow's milk* can result in the breakdown of these natural protective factors.

PHYSIOLOGY OF LACTATION (Fig. 1.4)

Two factors governed by hormones are involved in the physiology of lactation.

1. Production of milk
(prolactin)

Prolactin, a hormone secreted by the anterior pituitary gland, is essential for the production of breast milk but although its levels in the maternal circulation rise during pregnancy its action is blocked by the placental hormones. With separation and expulsion of the placenta at the end of labour, the oestrogen and progesterone levels are gradually reduced to the point where prolactin can be released and activated.

An increased blood supply circulates through the breast and essential substances for milk formation are extracted. Fatty globules and protein molecules from within the base of the secretory cells distend the acini and push their way into the lactiferous tubules.

Raised levels of prolactin inhibit ovulation and therefore have a contraceptive function as well, but the mother needs to breast feed 2- to 3-hourly for this to be fully effective. Prolactin levels are at

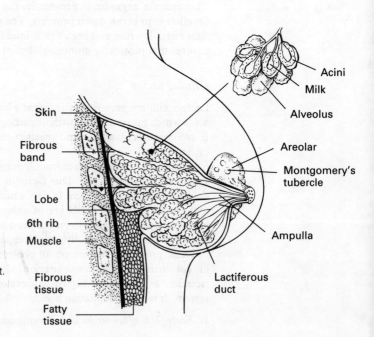

Fig. 1.4 The lactating breast. **Inset:** Proliferation and enlargement of alveoli showing degeneration of central granular tissue.

Acini
Milk
Alveolus
Skin
Fibrous band
Areolar
Montgomery's tubercle
Lobe
6th rib
Muscle
Ampulla
Fibrous tissue
Fatty tissue
Lactiferous duct

their highest during the night and if night feeds are the first to be discontinued – which they usually are – then more reliable methods of contraception must be used if pregnancy is to be avoided (see Ch. 11, p. 156 ff.).

2. Passage of milk
(oxytocin)

Two factors are involved in the transit of milk from the secretory cells to the nipple.

a. Back pressure

The force of new globules forming in the cells pushes the foremost ones into the lactiferous tubules and suckling the infant stimulates secretion of more milk.

b. Neurohormonal reflex
(let-down reflex)

When the baby is put to the breast, the rhythmical sucking movement produces nervous stimuli which cause an unconditioned reflex in the posterior pituitary gland. The direct result of this is the liberation of oxytocin from the posterior pituitary; this causes the **myoepithelial cells** ('basket' or 'spider' cells) around the alveoli to contract and push milk into the lactiferous vessels and so more milk flows to the ampullae. This 'let-down' reflex can be inhibited by pain, e.g. perineal sutures. It is therefore important to ensure that the mother is in a comfortable position, relaxed and pain-free, especially during feeding times.

This same oxytocic secretion also causes the uterine muscles to contract and so aids involution of that organ during the puerperium (Fig. 1.5).

Maintenance of lactation

Supply is maintained in response to demand. If the infant is not put to the breast, the milk supply will not be initiated. If a mother of twins puts both infants to the breast, the supply will be adequate for the two infants. The more often the infant is put to the breast, the better will be the milk supply.

Two factors are essential for the maintenance of lactation.

1. *Stimulus*
2. *Complete emptying of the breast.*

Stimulus

Breast fed babies need to feed frequently, especially in the early neonatal days. It is essential that the infant is 'fixed' at the breast correctly if he is to promote the right amount of stimulus. The stimulus of the infant's gums should be on the skin of the areola so

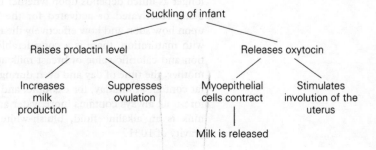

Fig. 1.5 Physiology of lactation

that pressure is exerted on the underlying ampullae where the milk is stored. It is therefore the breast from which he feeds – not the nipple. If mother complains of pain then the infant is not 'fixed' correctly.

In response to suckling, prolactin is released from the anterior pituitary gland and thus stimulates the manufacture of more milk. If for some reason the infant cannot feed from the breast initially, then the mother may express milk from her breast by hand or it may be initiated with a breast pump. However, the suckling of the infant provides much greater stimulus than either of these methods.

'Fixing' the infant (i.e. correct apposition of the infant's tongue and gums to the mother's nipple and areolar) is an art which needs to be learned by students before they attempt to help new mothers. Mother, baby and teaching midwife all need to find a comfortable position to achieve this end and may need to try different experimental positions.

Complete emptying of the breast The infant should empty one breast before being offered the second. If he does not empty the second breast then he should be offered that first at the next feed. Alternatively, he may be fed completely from one breast, the breasts then being used alternately for feeds. If the baby is to be really satisfied he needs both fore-milk and hind-milk at the same feed. This can only be achieved by the *complete* emptying of one breast.

It is important that the infant is fed whenever he wants and for as long as he wants so that supply is neither inadequate nor too great. If milk is not removed as it is produced, lactation may be suppressed because milk engorgement of the alveoli occurs and the 'basket' cells cannot contract. Milk cannot then be forced into the lactiferous ducts. It cannot be emphasised too strongly that feeding 'on demand' and stripping of the breast at each feed is also essential for the maintenance of lactation. Routines and patterns of feeding will be established and feeds will be less frequent when lactation is fully established.

COMPOSITION OF BREAST MILK

There is a gradual change from colostrum to 'mature' milk during the first 14 days of life. Sometimes this transitional phase takes even longer as much depends upon whether the glandular breast tissue is being reactivated or activated for the first time. It also depends upon how soon and how effectively the infant learns to suckle. Even with maturation, there is a considerable variation in the composition and calorific value of breast milk according to each individual mother, the time of day and even during one feed. There is a higher fat content at midday, for example, and in the hind-milk, while the fore-milk always contains more water and protein. The later breast milk is an alkaline fluid, bluish-white in colour with a specific gravity of 1031.

An average sample of breast milk, collected over 24 hours, is said to contain:

Protein 1.5%   Mineral salts 0.2%
Fat 3.5%   Water 87.8%
Carbohydrate 7.0%   Vitamins as in colostrum
Calorific value = 80 kilojoules per 30 ml.

Protein is much easier for the infant to digest than the protein in cow's milk. The curd protein is **casein**. Levels of the whey proteins, **lactalbumin** and **lactoglobulin**, are proportionally higher in breast milk than in cow's milk.

Fat Breast milk has equal proportions of saturated and unsaturated fats which the infant absorbs more easily than the coarse fat globule of cow's milk. The level of cholesterol is higher than in cow's milk. It is believed that, because the infant learns to deal with cholesterol at this early stage, there is a lower incidence of heart disease in adult life.

Carbohydrate contains the bifidus factor which is absent in cow's milk (see colostrum).

Mineral salts *Sodium* is at an ideal level for the human infant

Calcium
Phosphorus } more suitable for the infant than the higher levels
Magnesium   in cow's milk

Iron The low levels of iron do not reduce the anti-infective properties of lactoferrin (see colostrum).

Vitamins Levels of vitamins A, B, C, D and E are higher than in cow's milk but there is less vitamin K. Some paediatricians therefore give an injection of vitamin K to all newborn infants but this is not a universally accepted procedure.

Protective factors are present in breast milk as well as in colostrum:

- Protective immunoglobulins
- Lactoferrin
- Lysosome
- Antitrypsin factor
- Bifidus factor

THE PROMOTION OF BREAST FEEDING

Awareness of attitudes There are some adolescents and young women in our modern society who regard the breast more as a sex symbol than as a functional organ. It is valued as a means of attracting a male partner but its function as a means by which an infant is nourished scarcely enters their heads. This is not a criticism of their attitude but of the way in which we have reared and educated them.

Other women, recognising the function of the breast, nevertheless fear that, if breast feeding is established and prolonged for months, the shape and firmness of their breasts will be so affected that their sexual attractiveness will be lost.

Similarly, there are some husbands who admit quite honestly that they do not want their wives to breast feed. Pride in the wife's appearance and possible jealousy of the infant at the breast are two reasons often expressed.

To some career women, there is the added anxiety that breast feeding an infant for 4–6 months will interfere with professional and social activities and will perhaps be detrimental to promotion prospects. These are largely problems which have developed with our Western culture and they are very real to those women faced with them.

In an ideal world preparation for successful breast feeding would begin not only with each infant being successfully breast fed, but would continue as children observed their mother breast feeding younger brothers and sisters and happily weaning them. They would learn not only that 'breast is best' but that 'breast is normal'. It would begin with all children being reared by loving parents in a secure and caring home environment with the development of happy infantile, childhood and adolescent relationships. A woman who has personally experienced such 'parenting' and who accepts unequivocally her own sexual identity is much more likely to express her own intention to breast feed her children and also to succeed.

Unfortunately, we do not live in an ideal world! Many of today's pregnant women have never seen a baby being breast fed, and although breast feeding may be a natural function, in our society it is far from instinctive and is a technique which needs to be learned. Unfortunately, our own attitudes also brush off on newly arrived immigrant women who then query whether 'breast really is best' or not.

Education   Many local education authorities now have more enlightened teaching programmes which include 'Education for Living' modules to supplement academic subjects. Whenever and wherever possible, midwives should surely accept the opportunity to participate in these 'Health Education', GCSE Child Care courses and 'Preparation for Parenthood' classes which are now held in many schools and Colleges of Further Education. There can be a valuable interchange of thoughts and ideas with these young people, the next generation of parents. Above all, listen to them, be sensitive to the things they do **not** say; encourage the expression of their ideas and reactions, help them to verbalize their inhibitions and emotions. Whenever possible let them meet a newly delivered mother and her baby and discuss her attitudes towards him – especially in relation to breast feeding. Young people's attitudes can be greatly influenced by a well prepared and planned visit to a postnatal ward where they can talk freely with mothers who are successfully breast feeding. The visit will also help to dispel a popular misconception –

that the breasts miraculously fill with an abundance of freely flowing milk which runs easily into a baby's mouth whenever he opens it.

Emotional factors   To be breast fed is a baby's birthright. It gives him a feeling of security and a good foundation for the development of all personal relationships. To his mother it should bring that sense of final achievement which is the culmination of childbearing. Dr Frank Lake, a psychiatrist, described the awareness of '**BEING**' which arises in an infant in response to the relationship which develops between him and the attentive, loving mother who is able to meet his needs. This feeling of dependency in the early days of life is a fundamental human need. The infant needs to live in the 'light of his mother's countenance'.

He said that the denial of this response or its undue delay leads to an **ANXIETY OF SEPARATION** from **BEING** and personality problems throughout life; that the fulfilment of **WELL-BEING** becomes operative as the mother continues to give of her very self and to sustain her infant's needs during the first months of life. From such well-being there dawns in the infant a joyful self-consciousness and the development of status as a **PERSON** who is loved and satisfied. This is the way to normal independence, self security and self motivation. It is the foundation for outgoing and mature relationships in later life. The emotionally healthy person who has been aware of his **BEING** from his earliest days, who has lived in an atmosphere of loving relationships will thus be sustained in adult life during times of stress.

Mothers who feed their babies artificially need particularly to be aware of these facts and encouraged to hold their babies close when giving bottle feeds. They should try not to delegate the task to another member of the family, and remember that the bottle should be offered as though it were the breast. But they must never be made to feel guilty that they are unable to offer the breast.

The midwife then has a very difficult task when attempting to promote breast feeding. She is aware that 'breast is best', but must never put a mother under pressure to breast feed nor make her feel guilty if she bottle feeds. She must give enough guidance and support without being dogmatic or intrusive, yet she must give enough teaching and advice so that the mother does not feel inadequate or that she has been left to flounder.

FURTHER ADVANTAGES OF BREAST FEEDING

Less risk of   Milk taken directly from the breast by the infant is less likely to be
contamination   contaminated by pathogenic organisms and the incidence of neonatal infections is thus reduced.

In an age when dangers of contamination from radioactive fallout are much discussed, it should be brought to notice that breast milk contains far less strontium-90 than cow's milk.

Protection

The protective factors present in colostrum and breast milk have already been mentioned, namely, immunoglobulins, lactoferrin, lysosome, the bifidus factor and the antitrypsin factor. In particular, the incidence of gastroenteritis is very much reduced in breast-fed infants. The protective function of the immunoglobulins in relation to allergic conditions has also been mentioned. Where there is a family history of diseases such as asthma and eczema there is an even greater necessity for the mother to consider breast feeding.

Composition

Human milk provides food constituents in the correct balance for human growth. Cow's milk, on the other hand, must be modified in many ways before it can be tolerated by a human infant, whose rate of growth is much slower than that of the calf. Babies fed on cow's milk tend to gain weight much more quickly than those who are breast fed but such weight gain does not necessarily indicate healthy progress.

There is still some thought that certain babies have an intolerance to the protein in cow's milk and that the inhalation of milk following regurgitation can result in 'cot death'. This point might be mentioned at parentcraft classes but should not be used to frighten nervous mothers and coax them into breast feeding against their inclination. Neither should it be regarded as the only possible causes of cot death.

Convenience

Time and money can be saved by breast feeding. Feeds do not require preparation, expensive formula food does not have to be bought, nor is there any need to buy costly equipment which also needs to be cleaned and sterilised.

Physical factors

The neurohormonal reflex resulting in the let-down of milk has already been described. The oxytocin released during this reflex action also stimulates uterine contractions and so aids involution of the uterus.

The histological appearance of the secretory structures of the breast varies considerably with the duration of the lactation period and whether lactation has been suppressed, rather than initiated. The effects upon breast tissue of suppressing lactation are still not clear, but that the structures are affected is quite certain. With the tendency of our society to suppress lactation in its early weeks, or even to suppress its initiation, these tissue changes, and a possible increased risk of carcinoma of the breast, need to be borne in mind.

It has been shown that the current practice of allowing the infant to feed when he wishes and for as long as he wishes results in higher levels of prolactin circulating in the maternal bloodstream. It seems that these elevated levels suppress ovulation at least while the infant is being fully breast fed, (i.e. night feeding as well as full day feeding). It thus provides a natural method of contraception. However it is only 100% effective when the infant is suckling both by day and night and it is more usual to advise other contraceptive measures.

ANTENATAL CARE

Nutrition It is not necessary to make any great change in dietary habits if the expectant mother is already a well-nourished woman eating a well-balanced diet, but the antenatal clinic provides an excellent opportunity for revising the diet of those women who do not eat sensibly. An increase in the daily intake of protein is advised by many dieticians and also of calcium, a mineral which is stored in preparation for lactation. Iron is also stored to supply the infant's needs while he is being breast fed and therefore the mother's diet should contain daily some foods which contain this mineral. Additional iron, given with folic acid, is prescribed during pregnancy by some obstetricians but there is no general ruling about taking this. Vegans and some vegetarians may need extra counselling regarding their diet during pregnancy.

Examination Examination of the breasts will be carried out at the first antenatal visit as part of the general examination, and the breasts should be palpated in order to exclude any mass. Signs of pregnancy include greater venous prominence and pigmentation changes and the presence of Montgomery's tubercles should be noted.

To ask a mother at this stage if she plans to breast feed may well make her feel that she is being coerced into making a decision for which she is not yet ready. Should she herself broach the subject, then she will welcome time for discussion. Current research has exploded many long-held myths relating to the size and elasticity of the breasts and nipples, skin tone, texture, pigmentation and eversion of the nipples. There appears to be no evidence that any of these factors have any influence on successful lactation.

In particular, it is now agreed that an early examination of the nipple is of little use since, during the course of pregnancy and particularly towards the end, rising hormone levels result not only in pigmentation changes but in a greater eversion of the nipple. Even the inverted nipple may undergo a dramatic change. However, where a nipple is found to be inverted the mother should be asked if it has always been so. The midwife must bear in mind the possibility of carcinoma.

Records also need to be made in relation to breast surgery. The removal of breast cysts should cause no problem with the establishment of lactation, but following certain methods of mammoplasty or repositioning of the nipple, breast feeding may be impossible.

If the mother expresses a definite desire to breast feed then the midwife should record this fact on the mother's notes. She should also record whether the mother has breast fed any previous infants and the duration of lactation. If any problems arose, then they should be listed.

Hygiene Ordinary daily hygiene is all that is necessary. The use of soap on the nipple and areola should be avoided since most soaps will destroy the natural protective oils secreted by Montgomery's tubercles.

Support The majority of women feel more comfortable wearing a brassiere. Because the size and weight of the breasts increase during pregnancy, the midwife may be asked for advice concerning a suitable design. It is possible to obtain a brassiere which will expand up to 10 cm and can therefore be worn throughout pregnancy. As it has a front fastening it is also suitable for wearing in the lactation period. For comfort, it has wide shoulder straps and a deep diaphragm band. The advertised 'nursing' brassiere which has 'let-down' flaps should not be worn since it causes a ring of pressure around the breast. Some women also like to wear a night brassiere as their breasts become heavier.

Education Parentcraft classes always include a module relating to infant feeding and towards the end of pregnancy, in the last trimester, is probably the most effective time.

Information regarding the anatomy of the breast, physiology of lactation, initiation of lactation and demand feeding should all be discussed and questions relating to problems should be openly discussed. This is of particular importance when there are newly-arrived immigrant women in the class since our attitudes sometimes confuse them, leading them to believe that artificial feeding is a more accepted practice in modern society. The advantages of breast feeding over bottle feeding need to be stressed but the midwife must not be forceful or dogmatic in putting forward her point of view. Suitable literature should be available for the mothers to take away.

Well-planned teaching sessions in the postnatal ward can be very valuable if only two or three mothers are taken at a time. There they should be given the opportunity not just to talk with newly-delivered mothers whom they have met in the clinic and at classes, but to watch successful (but previously arranged) breast feeding as well.

At this stage, or after delivery and before discharge from hospital, information regarding support organisations such as the National Childbirth Trust and the Association of Breast Feeding Mothers will bring the realisation that there is a wealth of help available. The mother should also be aware that continual help from a midwife is available for all newly-delivered mothers, whether breast-feeding or not, for the first 28 days of her infant's life, and that a health visitor will continue to offer help if she requires it.

POSTNATAL CARE

General health The mother who is in good health, having had a normal labour and delivery, and who has been adequately prepared mentally and physically for breast feeding during the antenatal period, begins the lactation phase with every advantage. Her general health should be maintained and anaemia prevented at this time by the same well-balanced diet that she was eating prior to delivery. If she was taking iron antenatally it should be continued.

Adequate rest and avoidance of worry are extremely important factors, and the atmosphere surrounding the mother should be kept as tranquil as possible. Anxiety is not now believed to affect the neurohormonal reflex but a happy atmosphere is more conducive to successful lactation and good mother–baby bonding. Tiredness is underestimated as a contributory factor to the failure of breast feeding.

Support   As with antenatal women, most mothers feel more comfortable wearing a brassiere, especially on the 2nd and 3rd days when the breasts begin to fill. The type described for wearing during pregnancy is just as suitable postnatally. As colostrum or milk may leak from the breasts, disposable, absorbent pads can be worn inside the cups.

Hygiene   Ordinary daily hygiene as in the antenatal period.

Feeding technique   Following normal labour and delivery the baby should be put to the breast in the labour ward. If labour has not been normal then it should be done as soon as the condition of mother and baby allows. There can be no definite ruling about this, but in these early hours the mother normally longs to cuddle her baby to her breast and to feed him. There is little fluid in the breast so soon after delivery but the infant's instinctive sucking reflex should be satisfied too. The first few feeds should be enjoyed by mother and baby and should be assisted by a skilled midwife who can teach the mother how to 'fix' the infant correctly. Ward staff should be enthusiastic and united in their approach to breast feeding programmes. The infant should be fed whenever he appears hungry and for as long as he wishes. The mother should ensure that he empties the first breast before being offered the other. If the second breast is not emptied, then he should be offered that one first at the next feed.

Prolactin levels rise in proportion to the frequency of suckling. The more frequently the infant suckles, the more quickly will the transition from colostrum to true milk take place. As suckling also stimulates the production of oxytocin, so the more quickly will the neurohormonal reflex be established. The infant should also be breast fed by the mother at night rather than being given supplementary feeds so as not to disturb her. Milk production continues at night, when prolactin levels are at their highest, and if the breast is not emptied then the alveoli become congested and milk engorgement occurs. The fact that milk is produced in response to demand, and that successful lactation is largely dependent upon the efficient emptying of the breast as milk is produced, bears repetition yet again here.

Daily examination   Daily examination of the breast and nipples to assess milk flow and quantity and to exclude infection provides an opportunity to plan feeds during the next 24 hours.

Encouragement and assistance available to the mother at all times strengthen and support the other factors which are important for successful lactation:

- *Early initiation of feeding*
- *Correct positioning* of the infant at the mother's breast
- *Unrestricted duration and frequency* of feeding.

When she is discharged home, she should know whom to contact if she feels in need of help.

Suppression of lactation   If to be carried out immediately following delivery, then obviously the infant is not put to the breast in the labour ward. If there is no suckling, then the release of prolactin is not stimulated. On the 3rd or 4th day following delivery, engorgement of the blood vessels produces milk engorgement in the lactiferous vessels but milk should be expressed only very gently and *only* to relieve discomfort. The breasts should be well supported with a brassiere or breast binder while lactation is being suppressed. Discomfort can be relieved by the administration of a mild analgesic.

Drugs

Synthetic oestrogens   Can be used to depress the release of prolactin and so inhibit lactation but they are believed to increase the risk of embolism and carcinoma of the breast and are rarely used today.
Bromocriptine   Inhibits the release of prolactin. 2.5 mg is given on the first day and then 2.5 mg b.d. for 14 days.

These mothers are likely to start ovulating earlier than the mother who is breast feeding her infant and therefore need contraceptive advice. A low dosage progesterone-only 'pill' is commonly prescribed from the 7th postnatal day. It must be taken at the same time each day or it is not a reliable method.

REVISION QUESTIONS

Describe the anatomy of the female breast. What changes take place in the breasts during pregnancy?

Describe the female breast. What steps can be taken to assist successful breast feeding?

Describe the anatomy of the breast. Tabulate the indications and contraindications for breast feeding.

What can be done during pregnancy and after delivery to help the establishment of breast feeding?

Describe the changes which take place in the breast during pregnancy. What anatomical defects of the breast make breast feeding difficult? How would you deal with these?

Describe the anatomy of the female breast. Discuss the management of excessive fullness of the breasts in the early days of lactation.

Describe the anatomy of the breasts. What changes take place during pregnancy? What advice can be given to the expectant mother in preparation for successful breast feeding?

Describe the anatomy of the breast. Mrs P., a primigravida, wishes to breast feed her baby. What advice would you give her antenatally? What advice and support will she need postnatally?

Outline the physiology of lactation. Discuss the advantages of breast feeding. How, in the prenatal period, can mothers be encouraged to breast feed?

Discuss the advice and help a midwife should give to parents to assist in the establishment of infant feeding.

Describe how the midwife assists a woman to gain confidence and competence in her new role as a mother during the postnatal period.

What is the composition of human breast milk? How should cow's milk be modified to make it suitable for the neonate? What are the advantages of breast feeding?

What problems of breast feeding may occur during the early weeks of lactation? What advice and practical help can a midwife give to a woman experiencing difficulty with breast feeding?

Outline the role of the midwife in preparing a primigravida for breast feeding. Discuss the factors which influence: a) successful breast feeding; b) discontinuation of breast feeding.

What care and advice may be given to a primigravida by the midwife to promote and support successful breast feeding: a) during pregnancy; b) in the first 10 days after the birth? What help is available to a mother who is breast feeding once she has been discharged from the midwife's care?

How may the midwife help the mother to establish breast feeding successfully when her baby is receiving care in an incubator?

Give: two essential factors required for breast feeding
three advantages of breast feeding
one disadvantage of breast feeding.

REFERENCES AND FURTHER READING

Books and reports

Cirket C 1989 A woman's guide to breast health. Grapevine, Wellingborough

Dana N, Price A 1991 Working woman's guide to breast feeding. Meadowbrook Press, Deephaven, MN

Department of Health and Social Security 1976 Breast feeding. Nutrition Information Bulletin Nos 126 and 127. Her Majesty's Stationery Office, London

Department of Heath and Social Security 1988 Present day practice in infant feeding. Health and Social Subjects No 32. Her Majesty's Stationery Office, London

Klaus M H, Kennell J H 1982 Parent–infant bonding, 2nd edn. C V Mosby, St Louis

Lake F 1986 Clinical theology: a theological and psychological basis to clinical pastoral care. Darton, Longman & Todd, London

Llewellyn-Jones D 1983 Breast feeding – how to succeed: questions and answers for mothers. Faber & Faber, London

Messenger M 1982 The breastfeeding book. Century, London

Raphael D 1979 Breastfeeding and food policy in a hungry world. International Conference on Human Lactation, New York, 1977. Academic Press, New York

Royal College of Midwives 1991 Successful breast feeding. Churchill Livingstone, Edinburgh

Stern D N 1977 The first relationship: infant and mother. Fontana, London

Thomas P Encourage the mother. Association of Breast-feeding Mothers, London

Articles

Anderson E, Geden E 1991 Nurses' knowledge of breastfeeding. Journal of Obstetrical, Gynecological and Neonatal Nursing 20(1): 58–64

Angerbach K 1990 Breast feeding fallacies. Their relationship to understanding lactation. Birth 17(1): 44–49

Beck M 1989 Breast feeding: the midwife's role. Midwives' Chronicle 102: 412–413

Davies R 1988 Postnatal care and breast feeding. Practitioner 232: 1271–1272

Dicken A 1991 Counselling when breast feeding is not possible. New Generation (March): 32–33

Dwyer R 1991 Breast feeding and birth control. Lancet 337: 1415

Eaton J 1991 Breast feeding. Suppressing lactation. Nursing Times 87(18): 27–30

Elstein M 1968 Physiology of lactation. Midwife and Health Visitor (May)

Fisher C 1981 Breast feeding. A midwife's view. Maternal and Child Health (Feb): 52–57

Fisher C 1983 Positions of success. New Generation 2(3): 20–21

Fisher C 1984 The initiation of breast feeding. Midwives' Chronicle 97: 39–41

Fisher C 1984 Baby knows best. Senior Nurse (July): 12

Gray RH, Campbell O M, Apelo R, Eslami S S, Zacur H, Ramos R M, Gehret J C, Labbok M H 1990 Risk of ovulation during lactation. Lancet 335: 25–29

Henschel D 1990 The joint breast feeding initiative. Midwives' Chronicle 103: 284

Howie P et al 1980 The relationship between suckling-induced prolactin response and lactogenesis. Journal of Clinical Endocrinology and Metabolism 50: 670–673

Howie P et al 1980 The initiation of lactation. Midwife, Health Visitor and Community Nurse 16 (April): 142–147

Howie P et al 1985 Breast feeding: a new understanding. Midwives' Chronicle 98: 184–192

Howie P et al 1990 Protective effect of breast feeding against infection. British Medical Journal 300: 11–16

Humenick S 1987 Clinical significance of breast feeding maturation rates. Birth 14(4): 174

Inch S 1991 Furthering the aims of the JBI locally. Midwives' Chronicle 104: 172–173

Jordan P, Wall V 1990 Breast feeding and fathers. Birth 17(4): 210–213

Kearney M 1988 Identifying psycho-social obstacles to breast feeding success. Journal of Obstetrical, Gynecological and Neonatal Nursing 17(2): 98–105

Kremer J A 1990 Lactation inhibition by a single injection of a new depot bromocriptine. British Journal of Obstetrics and Gynaecology 97(6): 527–532

Levi J 1991 Breast feeding: common problems and solutions. RCGP Connection (May): 2–3

McNeilly A S et al 1982 Fertility after childbirth: pregnancy associated with breast feeding. Clinical Endocrinology 18: 169–173

Minchin M 1989 Positioning for breast feeding. Birth 16(2): 67–74
Newton C 1991 When do women decide to breast feed? Nursing Times
  87(2): 49
Purves L 1990 What are fathers for? Parents (June): 34–35
Salariya E M et al 1978 Duration of breast feeding after early initiation and
  frequent feeding. Lancet ii: 1141–1143
Thomson A 1989 Breast feeding: a contraceptive. Midwifery 5(3): 105
Wolf F 1991 Breast feeding and birth control (letter). Lancet 337: 911
Woolridge M W 1986 The anatomy of infant suckling. Midwifery
  2(4): 164–171

Voluntary societies that promote breast feeding
Association of Breast Feeding Mothers, 131 Mayow Road, London SE26
  (Tel. 081-778-4769)
La Leche League, B M 3424, London WC1V 6XX (Tel. 081-404-5011)
National Childbirth Trust Breast Feeding Promotion Group, 9
  Queensborough Terrace, London W2 3TB (071-221-3822)

2 The female pelvis

Situation	The pelvis articulates with the 5th lumbar vertebra above and with the heads of the right and left femur in the corresponding acetabulum. The weight of the trunk is transmitted through the pelvis to the legs.
Shape	It is similar to a bony basin, which is what its name implies, and it forms a girdle to give protection to the pelvic organs.
Size	It is the largest formation of bone in the body.
Gross structure (Fig. 2.1)	It is composed of four bones: • the *sacrum* • the *coccyx* • two *innominate bones*
The sacrum	is formed by the fusion of five sacral vertebrae. It is triangular in shape with the apex pointing downwards and lies like a wedge between the right and left innominate bones with which it articulates. Four pairs of foraminae are formed where the vertebrae fuse and these communicate with the sacral canal. Through the foraminae, nerves from the spinal cord pass, together with blood

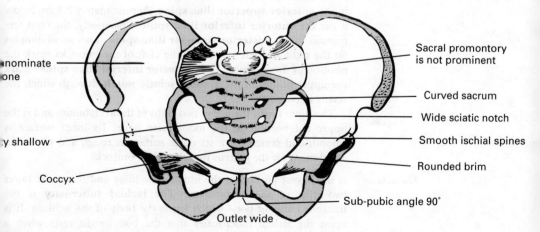

Innominate bone

Very shallow

Coccyx

Outlet wide

Sub-pubic angle 90°

Sacral promontory is not prominent

Curved sacrum

Wide sciatic notch

Smooth ischial spines

Rounded brim

Fig. 2.1 Normal female pelvis.

vessels and lymphatics. The sacrum forms the posterior wall of the pelvic cavity.

The **hollow of the sacrum** is the concave anterior surface of the sacrum. This concavity helps to increase the capacity of the true pelvis.

The **alae** (sing. **ala**) are the widened-out wings of bone on each side of the 1st sacral vertebra.

The **promontory** is the centre point of the upper border of the first sacral vertebra which, with the base of the 5th lumbar vertebra, protrudes over the hollow of the sacrum.

The **sacral canal** runs longitudinally through the centre of the sacrum and opens at the level of the 5th sacral vertebra. It forms a passage for the spinal nerves, which fan out at the level of the 2nd and 3rd sacral vertebrae to form the **cauda equina**. During labour, some obstetricians introduce local anaesthetic into the caudal canal as a means of relieving the pain of uterine contractions. The nerves below the 2nd sacral vertebra are temporarily paralysed although the patient remains fully conscious and able to co-operate.

The coccyx   Four fused vertebrae make up this tiny bone, which is triangular in shape with its base lying uppermost and articulating with the sacrum. Muscles and ligaments are attached to its tip.

Right and left innominate bones (Fig. 2.2)   The sacrum forms a wedge between the right and left innominate bones which lie on each side of it. In the adult the innominate bone appears to be one large irregular-shaped bone, but before the age of 25 years it is not completely ossified and is actually made up of bones which develop from three primary centres of ossification.

The three parts are named the ilium, ischium and pubis. They meet in the cup-shaped depression which is known as the **acetabulum**.

The ilium   is surmounted by the **iliac crest**, which can be palpated quite easily if the hands are placed on the hips. The crest terminates anteriorly in the **anterior superior iliac spine**. Approximately 2.5 cm below it lies the **anterior inferior iliac spine**. Posteriorly, the crest terminates in the **posterior superior iliac spine**. Two small dimples on the right and left just above the cleft of the buttocks mark the position of these spines. The **posterior inferior iliac spines** mark the upper border of the **greater sciatic notch** through which the sciatic nerve passes.

The ilium forms the upper two-fifths of the acetabulum and is the upper flat portion of the innominate bone. Its inner surface is smooth and concave but its outer surface is rough and makes an attachment for the gluteus muscles of the buttocks.

The ischium   is the lowest portion of the innominate bone and forms the lower two-fifths of the acetabulum. The **ischial tuberosity** is the thickened area of bone which forms the body of the ischium. It is upon the ischial tuberosities that the bodyweight rests when a person is in the sitting position. The **ischial spine** lies approx-

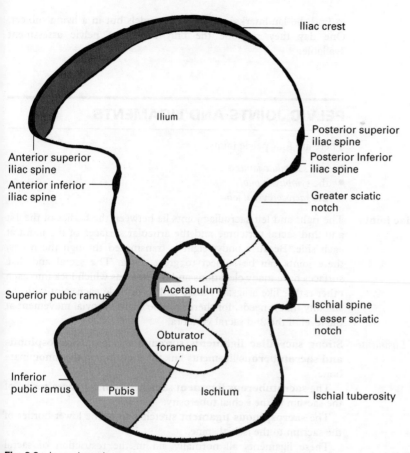

Fig. 2.2 Innominate bone.

The pubis

imately 2.5 cm above the ischial tuberosity and it divides the **greater and lesser sciatic notches**.

This is the smallest of the three components of the innominate bone and forms the lowest one-fifth of the acetabulum. The right and left pubic bones unite with each other anteriorly at the square-shaped pubic bodies. They are fused by a pad of cartilage, the **symphysis pubis**. Extending upwards from each pubic body, the **superior ramus** unites with the ilium at the **iliopectineal eminence**. The inferior ramus extends downwards to unite with the ischium. The **right and left inferior** (or **descending**) **rami** form the **pubic arch**. The foramen surrounded by the ischium and pubis is the **obturator foramen**.

Some of these landmarks may appear quite irrelevant to student midwives working in the UK. In remote areas of the Third World, where radiography and ultrasound machines are unlikely to be freely available, they really will be of practical use. Students should therefore make themselves aware of and recognise where to find the landmarks, not only on models but in a living subject. One day they may be the only means of pelvic assessment available.

PELVIC JOINTS AND LIGAMENTS

There are four pelvic joints:

- two *sacroiliac joints*
- the *symphysis pubis*
- the *sacrococcygeal joint*

Two sacroiliac joints The right and left sacroiliac joints lie between the bodies of the 1st and 2nd sacral vertebrae and the articular surfaces of the ilium at each side. Because bodyweight is transmitted through the pelvis, these joints can be subject to great strain. The sacral and iliac surfaces have many elevations and depressions which lock into each other rather like a jigsaw puzzle and so provide each joint with the stability that it needs, for there is some slight synovial movement at the level of the 2nd sacral vertebra.

Ligaments Strong **sacroiliac ligaments** surround the joint. **Sacrospinous and sacrotuberous** ligaments link the sacrum and the innominate bone.

The **sacrotuberous ligament** stretches from the lower border of the sacrum to the ischial tuberosity.

The **sacrospinous ligament** stretches from the lower border of the sacrum to the ischial spine.

These ligaments all normally aid in the restriction of sacral movement.

The symphysis pubis is a secondary cartilaginous joint approximately 4 cm in length. The articulating surfaces of the bodies of the pubic bones are covered with hyaline cartilage and a disc of fibrocartilage unites the two bodies. **Pubic ligaments** surround the joint and it has only minimal mobility.

The sacrococcygeal joint is also a secondary cartilaginous joint and is formed between the lower border of the sacrum and the upper border of the coccyx. It is surrounded and supported by **sacrococcygeal ligaments** and is capable of flexion and extension, movements which are passive during defaecation and labour.

Poupart's ligament, also known as the **inguinal ligament**, extends between the anterior superior iliac spine and the body of the pubis.

Obturator membrane: Except for a small space which allows the passage of blood vessels, nerves and lymphatics, the obturator membrane fills the obturator foramen.

These joints all increase their power of movement during pregnancy because a degree of laxity in their supporting ligaments is brought about by the hormone relaxin. Details relating to the pelvis during pregnancy and labour will be found later in the chapter.

DIVISIONS OF THE PELVIS

The **brim** of the pelvis divides it into two parts, the false and the true pelvis. The **false pelvis** lies above the pelvic brim and is of little importance in midwifery. The **true pelvis** includes the pelvic brim and all the area that lies below it. It is described as having a **brim**, a **cavity** and an **outlet** and forms the curved canal through which the fetus must pass to be born.

The brim or inlet (Fig. 2.3A)
This is almost round in shape in the normal female pelvis and eight points can be demonstrated on it:

1. The promontory of the sacrum
2. The ala of the sacrum
3. The sacroiliac joint
4. The iliopectineal line
5. The iliopectineal eminence
6. The inner border of the superior pubic ramus
7. The body of the pubic bone
8. The upper border of the symphysis pubis.

The cavity (Fig. 2.3B)
The cavity extends from the brim of the pelvis above to the pelvic outlet below. Formed by the **hollow of the sacrum**, the **posterior wall** is deeply concave and is approximately 10 cm in length. The **anterior wall** is formed by the **symphysis pubis** and is ap-

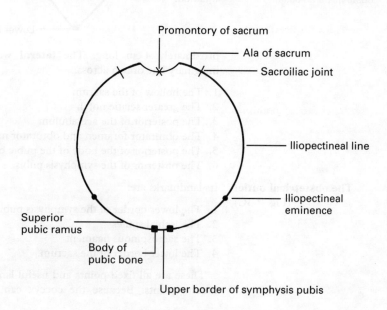

Fig. 2.3A Landmarks of pelvic brim.

Promontory of sacrum
Ala of sacrum
Sacroiliac joint
Iliopectineal line
Iliopectineal eminence
Superior pubic ramus
Body of pubic bone
Upper border of symphysis pubis

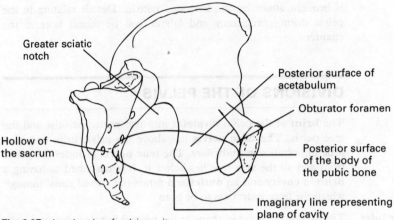

Fig. 2.3B Landmarks of pelvic cavity.

Greater sciatic notch

Posterior surface of acetabulum

Obturator foramen

Hollow of the sacrum

Posterior surface of the body of the pubic bone

Imaginary line representing plane of cavity

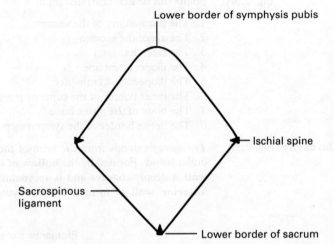

Lower border of symphysis pubis

Ischial spine

Fig. 2.3C Landmarks of obstetric pelvic outlet.

Sacrospinous ligament

Lower border of sacrum

proximately 4 cm long. The **lateral walls** are formed by an imaginary line drawn across:

1. The hollow of the sacrum
2. The greater sciatic notch
3. The posterior of the acetabulum
4. The obturator foramen and obturator membrane
5. The posterior of the body of the pubic bone
6. The posterior of the symphysis pubis.

The obstetrical outlet
(Fig. 2.3C)

Its landmarks are:

1. The lower border of the symphysis pubis
2. The ischial spines
3. The sacrospinous ligament
4. The lower border of the sacrum.

These are all fixed points and useful landmarks for taking pelvic measurements. Because the coccyx can tip backwards and the ligaments are capable of stretching, there is more room for the fetus to pass than is at first apparent. The available room is therefore known as the **obstetrical outlet**.

MEASUREMENTS OF THE PELVIS

The brim (Fig. 2.4A)

The distance between the promontory of the sacrum and the inner upper border of the symphysis pubis is known as the **antero-posterior diameter** (or **true conjugate**) and in the normal female pelvis it should not be less than 11 cm. The **oblique diameter** is the distance between the sacroiliac joint and the opposite iliopectineal eminence: it should not be less than 12 cm. Measured between the two widest points of the pelvic brim, the **transverse diameter** should measure at least 13 cm. (In the female pelvis this is right across the centre of the pelvic brim.) The measurement taken between the promontory of the sacrum and either ilio-pectineal eminence, which should be at least 9.5 cm, is known as the **sacrocotyloid diameter**.

The cavity (Fig. 2.4B)

The **anteroposterior diameter** is taken from the junction of the 2nd and 3rd sacral vertebrae to the midpoint of the symphysis pubis. The **oblique diameter** is measured at the same level in the pelvis as the anteroposterior diameter and runs parallel to the oblique diameter of the pelvic brim. There are no fixed points to measure between.

In theory, the **transverse diameter** is a measurement taken between the two points farthest apart on the lateral pelvic walls. As there are no fixed points in the cavity these measurements cannot be accurately assessed but, as the cavity is circular, all diameters must be equal and they should all be at least 12 cm.

The outlet (Fig. 2.4C)

Measured from the lower border of the symphysis pubis to the lower border of the sacrum, the **anteroposterior diameter** should measure not less than 13 cm. The **oblique diameter** is impossible to measure accurately because the sacrotuberous ligaments stretch when they are distended by the fetal head. Nevertheless, it is accepted as lying parallel to the oblique diameters of the brim and cavity and should be at least 12 cm. The **transverse diameter** is estimated between either the ischial tuberosities or the ischial spines (both measurements being the same in the normal pelvis); this diameter should be 11 cm at the minimum.

Two other measurements must be mentioned, the diagonal conjugate and the obstetrical conjugate. The **diagonal conjugate** can be assessed by vaginal examination and indicates the size of the pelvic brim. It is the distance between the lower border of the symphysis pubis and the promontory of the sacrum. The **obstetrical conjugate** is a measurement made between the inner surface, at the centre, of the symphysis pubis and the promontory of the sacrum.

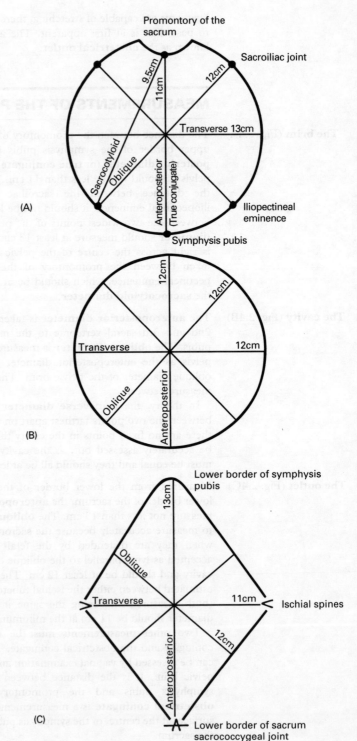

Fig. 2.4 Measurements of the pelvis (A) brim (B) cavity (C) outlet.

Table 2.1 Table of measurements

	AP	Oblique	Transverse
Brim	11 cm	12 cm	13 cm
Cavity	12 cm	12 cm	12 cm
Outlet	13 cm	12 cm	11 cm

Note: These measurements are accepted as being the normal minimum.

All these measurements can be made accurately only by X-ray pelvimetry. The minimal measurements of the normal European female pelvis have been recorded here, but measurements vary considerably among the different races and even among women of the same race. This must be remembered in the cosmopolitan populations of today. In recent years, it seems also that the size of the female pelvis has increased in all countries of the world.

PLANES OF THE PELVIS (Fig. 2.5)

The planes of the pelvis are imaginary flat surfaces drawn at the level of the brim, cavity and outlet. It has been shown that the planes are of differing size; therefore they must each also be of differing shape.

Plane of the brim

marks the boundary between the false and true pelvis.

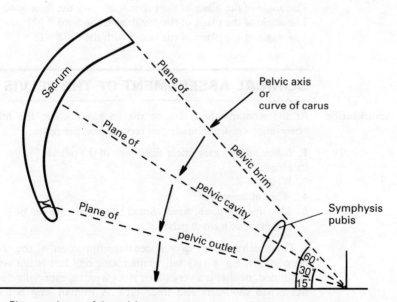

Fig. 2.5 Planes and axes of the pelvis.

Plane of the cavity

is the plane of the greatest pelvic dimensions – the most roomy part of the pelvis. It passes through the upper border of the 3rd sacral vertebra and the midpoint of the symphysis pubis.

Plane of the outlet

is the plane of the least pelvic dimensions. It passes through the lower border of the sacrum and the lower border of the symphysis pubis.

AXIS OF THE PELVIS

The **curve of Carus** is an imaginary line drawn at right angles to each of these planes and is said to be the **pelvic axis**, the path which the fetus takes as it travels through the birth canal. The line is drawn midway between the anterior and posterior walls of the pelvic cavity.

INCLINATION OF THE PELVIS

When a person is standing upright, the plane of the pelvic brim makes an angle of 60° with the floor. Because the pelvis is a curved canal, the angles of the brim, cavity and outlet must be different too, i.e.:

The angle of the plane of the pelvic brim with the floor = 60°
The angle of the plane of the cavity with the floor = 30°
The angle of the plane of the outlet with the floor = 15°

CLINICAL ASSESSMENT OF THE PELVIS

General examination At the woman's first visit to the antenatal clinic the following observations must be made and recorded on her notes:

1. *Ethnic origin* – may affect size/shape of the pelvis
2. *Height*
3. *Weight*
4. *Waist measurement*
5. *Shoe size* and *size of hands*. Small bone structure can be indicative of a small pelvis.

These observations give a general impression of the woman's proportions, e.g. a very tall woman with tiny feet is not well proportioned, neither is a very short, stout woman, especially if she also has broad shoulders and thick hips. A woman who is less than 1.50 cm tall is likely to have a small pelvis.

The student midwife must practise this observation and always be alert for the patient who walks with a limp or who has muscle wasting of the legs. These may give an indication of congenital hip deformity, anterior poliomyelitis, injury or other conditions which cause consequent pelvic deformities. This type of observation is especially important if, because of language difficulties, it is impossible to take a full medical history. Whenever possible, the woman should be asked if she has ever been involved in an accident or received injuries to her spine, pelvis or legs.

Obstetric history   A careful history should be taken of previous labours and deliveries. If the woman has previously had a normal labour and delivery following a 40-week gestation period, and if the infant weighed at least 3 kg, it may be accepted that her pelvis is of adequate size. Should she be a primigravida, not have delivered a fair-sized infant or perhaps have a previous history of instrumental delivery or caesarean section, then it cannot be assumed that her pelvis will be adequate and further observations and investigations become of vital importance.

External measurements   These are rarely used in countries where more accurate means of pelvic assessment are available, but are often used by midwives working alone in remote areas overseas. The measurements are by no means accurate but will give an approximate size and shape of the pelvis and reveal any gross disproportion. Three measurements are taken, using an instrument called a **pelvimeter**.

Interspinous diameter   The points of the pelvimeter are placed one over each anterior
(Fig. 2.6A)   superior iliac spine and the distance between them is normally 25.5 cm.

Intercristal diameter   The points of the pelvimeter are moved upwards over the iliac crests
(Fig. 2.6A)   and the measurement between the two widest points, usually about 28 cm, is recorded. There is normally a difference of 2.5 cm between these two diameters. If the difference is greater than 2.5 cm then a 'flat' pelvis which is contracted at the brim should be suspected.

External conjugate   The woman is turned to lie on her side. One point of the pelvimeter
(Fig. 2.6B)   is placed over the centre of the upper border of the symphysis pubis and the other point is placed over the tip of the spine of the 5th lumbar vertebra. This is found by marking a point between the two dimples made by the posterior superior iliac spines and then moving upwards for about 2.5 cm. This measurement is usually about 19 cm. To allow for subcutaneous tissues, 9 cm is subtracted and the resultant figure gives an estimation of the anteroposterior diameter of the brim.

Transverse diameter of the   No pelvimeter is necessary for the fourth assessment, the **trans-**
outlet   **verse of the outlet**. The woman lies in position as for vaginal examination. The midwife, wearing a glove, makes her hand into a fist and places it between the patient's ischial tuberosities. It should be possible for this diameter to admit the four knuckles of the

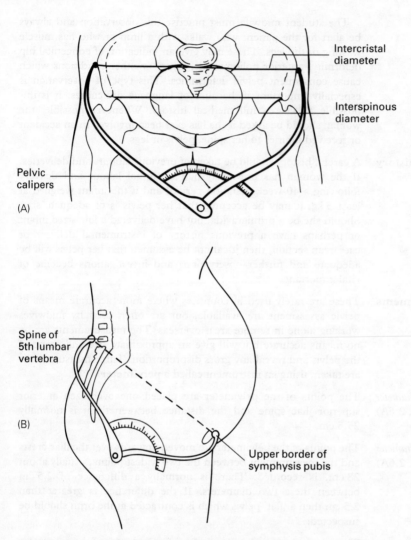

Fig. 2.6 (A) and (B) External measurements.

clenched fist. Each midwife should know the measurement of her own knuckles, usually 7.5–9 cm. Allowing for subcutaneous tissues, the actual measurement is therefore approximately 10–11.5 cm between these bony tuberosities.

Abdominal palpation A pelvis cannot be said to be adequate until the widest transverse diameter of the fetal head has passed through the pelvic brim. Once the head has passed through these bony borders, it should be able to pass through the cavity and the outlet, where some of the borders, being ligaments, are capable of distension. The only exception occurs when there is a contracted outlet, recognisable by sharp prominent ischial spines or by a narrow pubic arch.

It is therefore important that at the 36th–37th week of pregnancy, the abdomen is palpated to see if the fetal head is 'engaged' or can be made to 'engage', i.e. the widest transverse diameter of the fetal head can be pushed through the pelvic brim. If the fetal head cannot be made to engage, the woman should be seen by an obstetrician for this examination so that adequacy of the pelvis can be confirmed.

Engagement of the head
(Fig. 2.7)

To make this assessment on abdominal palpation, it is essential that:

1. The woman's bladder is empty
2. The upper margin of the symphysis pubis is defined
3. The levels of the occiput and of the sinciput are accurately defined.

Until fairly recently, the fetal head was either described as being 'engaged' or 'not engaged' but current practice is to estimate the degree of engagement in fifths.

Vaginal examination

In remote areas of the world where modern diagnostic techniques are not available, and unless there is a previous history of abortion, the doctor usually performs a vaginal examination on every new patient attending the antenatal clinic. This is not only to confirm the pregnancy but also to exclude abnormalities of the pelvis and its contents. A further examination is made at the 36th–37th week of pregnancy to ensure that the fetal head will pass through the pelvis and to assess the pelvic brim, cavity and outlet (Fig. 2.8A, B, C).

Assessment of the brim
(Fig. 2.8A)

If the head is not already through the pelvic brim, an assessment is made by estimating the diagonal conjugate. The two index fingers are placed in the vagina, running them immediately beneath the symphysis pubis and attempting to reach the promontory of the sacrum. The thumb is placed externally over the symphysis pubis. If the sacral promontory cannot be felt, then the diagonal conjugate, and therefore the brim of the pelvis, is said to be adequate. If the sacral promontory can be felt, then the diagonal conjugate is reduced in diameter and the doctor or rural midwife/birth attendant making this examination will refer the patient to a hospital consultant obstetrician for further investigations.

Assessment of the cavity
(Fig. 2.8B)

Only when the fetal head is not in the pelvis is it possible to feel the **curve of the sacrum**. It should be well hollowed and not straight. The **sacrospinous ligament** should then be sought. This should be the width of two fingers across the **greater sciatic notch**.

Assessment of the outlet
(Fig. 2.8C)

The fingers are run to the lateral borders of the outlet, feeling for the **ischial spines**, which should be well rounded and not sharp or projecting inwards.

The **pubic arch** should be well rounded so that two fingers can be placed in the angle of the arch. If this is not possible, then a narrow subpubic angle is diagnosed, limiting the room available at the outlet. Before completing this examination, the trans-

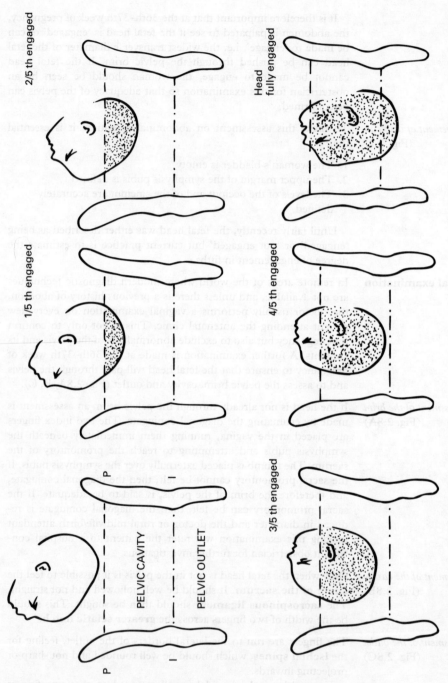

Fig. 2.7 Engagement of the fetal head assessed in fifths. PP (– – –) = pelvic brim, II (– · – ·) = ischial spines.

verse diameter of the outlet (mentioned previously) should be assessed.

These assessments are now almost obsolete practice in the UK.

X-ray pelvimetry   This is an accurate method of estimating the relationship between the maternal pelvis and fetal head.

Before the examination is carried out, the patient's bladder and rectum should both be emptied. A standing lateral picture is taken so that the radiologist can measure the anteroposterior diameters of the pelvic brim, cavity and outlet. These measurements are then compared with the size of the fetal skull. In consultation with the

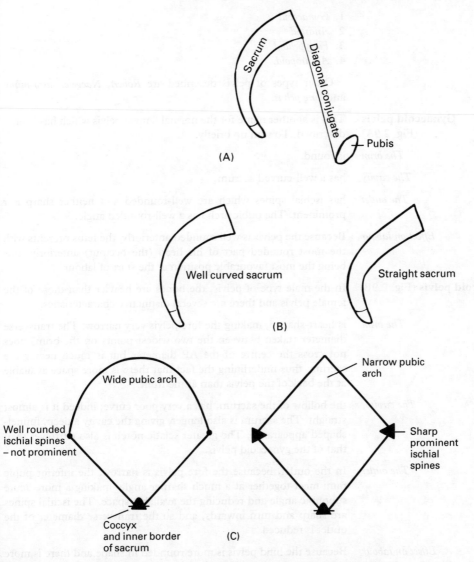

Fig. 2.8   Assessment of pelvis by vaginal examination: (A) brim (B) cavity (C) outlet.

radiologist, the obstetrician is then able to decide whether a vaginal delivery should be attempted or whether elective caesarean section must be carried out.

VARIETIES OF PELVIS

It is possible to tell the sex, and sometimes the race, of a person by the shape of the pelvis. The normal classification used is that of Caldwell and Molloy.

There are four main groups:

1. *Gynaecoid*
2. *Android*
3. *Platypelloid*
4. *Anthropoid.*

Other types of pelvis described are *Robert*, *Naegele*, *justo-minor* and *long pelvis.*

Gynaecoid pelvis (Fig. 2.9A) — This is another name for the normal female pelvis which has been described. To sum up briefly:

The brim — is round.

The cavity — has a well-curved sacrum.

The outlet — has ischial spines which are well-rounded and neither sharp nor prominent. The pubic arch has a well-rounded angle.

Effect on labour — Because the pelvis is well rounded anteriorly, the fetus presents with the most rounded part of his head (the occiput) anteriorly, this being the most favourable position at the start of labour.

Android pelvis (Fig. 2.9B) — In the male type of pelvis, the bones are heavier than those of the female pelvis and there are several distinctive characteristics.

The brim — is heart-shaped, making the fore pelvis very narrow. The transverse diameter (taken between the two widest points on the brim) does not cross the centre of the AP diameter but is much nearer the sacrum, thus underlining the fact that there is more space available at the back of the pelvis than at the front.

The cavity, — the hollow of the sacrum, has a very poor curve; indeed it is almost straight. The sacrum is also longer, giving the cavity a deep, funnel-shaped appearance. The greater sciatic notch is also narrower than that of the gynaecoid pelvis.

The outlet — In the outlet, because the fore pelvis is narrow, the inferior pubic rami meet together at a much sharper angle, making a more acute subpubic angle and reducing the available space. The ischial spines are sharp and turn inwards, and so the transverse diameter of the outlet is reduced.

Effect on labour (see also Ch. 15, p. 225 ff.) — Because the hind pelvis is more rounded in shape and there is more available space, the fetus lies with his occiput in the right or left posterior quadrant. In about 90% of such posterior positions, although labour tends to be prolonged, delivery is normal. Some of these normal deliveries will occur as persistent occipitoposterior positions (i.e. born face to pubes) while a smaller proportion will be face presentations.

However, a straight sacrum will prevent rotation of the fetal head, prominent ischial spines will prevent descent and a narrow pubic arch will not allow delivery of the occiput. In these instances there will be a need for manual rotation of the head and instrumental delivery or caesarean section.

Platypelloid pelvis
(Fig. 2.9C)

This may be due to developmental, rachitic or hereditary factors. It is often seen in African women, possibly due not only to poor dietary factors but to the custom of carrying heavy weights on the head during the developmental years.

The brim

has a short anteroposterior diameter but the transverse diameter is lengthened, giving the brim a kidney- or bean-shaped appearance.

The cavity

The diameters are affected in the same way as those of the brim but there is usually room for the fetal head.

The outlet

Because the pelvis is shallow, the inferior rami meet at a very gradual angle to form a very wide pubic arch, and therefore a capacious outlet.

The simple flat pelvis should also be described here. At the brim it resembles the rachitic pelvis, having a reduced anteroposterior diameter. Unlike the rachitic pelvis, however, the diameters of the cavity and outlet are smaller than normal.

Effect on labour
(see also p. 225 ff.)

The fetal head finds difficulty in engaging at the pelvic brim and usually presents with the long diameter of the head across the transverse diameter of the brim where most room is available. Because of the high head, the membranes will very likely rupture early and there is the possibility of cord prolapse.

The following occurrences are all possible outcomes of labour:

1.   With good uterine contractions, the head is pushed to and fro between the sacral promontory and the symphysis pubis. It then 'rocks and rolls' through the brim to the cavity. The skull bones overlap each other with this pressure, and the process is known as **asynclitism**. Rapid delivery of the head may then follow.

2.   The biparietal diameter of the fetal skull is held in the sacrocotyloid diameter of the pelvic brim, and uterine contractions cause the head to extend as it descends (normally, flexion occurs as the head descends). This results in a **face presentation**.

3.   If the brim is greatly contracted, the fetal head remains floating high above it and **caesarean section** becomes imperative. This is a fairly common occurrence in countries where there is very little antenatal care, but may be seen in the UK in a woman who has clinical signs of rickets. Caesarean section is then carried out before the patient goes into labour, exposing mother and infant to a lesser risk of traumatic injury.

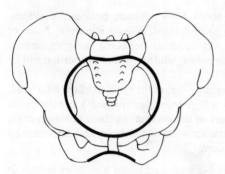

Fig. 2.9A Gynaecoid pelvis.

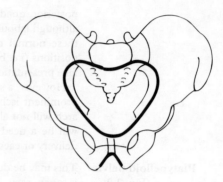

Fig. 2.9B Android pelvis.

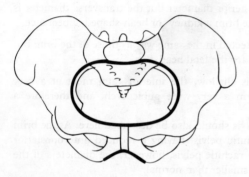

Fig. 2.9C Platypelloid pelvis.

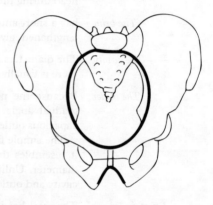

Fig. 2.9D Anthropoid pelvis.

Anthropoid pelvis (Fig. 2.9D)	Very tall, long-legged Caucasian women are frequently found to have this type of pelvis and it is quite common in the women of South Africa.
The brim	is oval-shaped, having a long anteroposterior diameter but a reduced transverse diameter.
The cavity	is adequate in all diameters but is rather deep.
The outlet	is adequate in all diameters, with the pubic arch being rather wide.
Effect on labour (see also p. 225 ff.)	The fetus commonly presents with the long diameter of the head in the anteroposterior diameter of the pelvic brim where it can be most easily accommodated. The occiput more often lies in the hollow of the sacrum rather than directly anterior. The fetus then passes through the pelvis, remaining in the same position, and delivers in the **unreduced occipitoposterior position** instead of face to perineum.
Long pelvis (Palfrey 1974)	In clinical practice Palfrey found a higher incidence of sacralisation of the lumbar vertebra than textbooks suggest. The effect on labour

is that of the anthropoid pelvis, i.e. a higher incidence of persistent occipitoposterior position and also of breech presentation.

Justo-minor pelvis   This is a miniature gynaecoid pelvis. It is truly gynaecoid in shape but all diameters are equally reduced. It is to be found in the petite woman who is less than 1.5 m tall. She may deliver a small baby vaginally with very little trouble. On the other hand, a larger baby may require a forceps delivery or even caesarean section.

Contracted pelvis   This is a pelvis in which one or more of the essential diameters (i.e. anteroposterior, oblique or transverse of brim, cavity or outlet) is reduced by 1 cm or more.

These then are the main categories of pelvis, but it must be remembered that the majority of abnormalities cannot be clearly defined as belonging to one of these groups. Most abnormal pelves have just one of these varying attributes.

The **straight sacrum** associated with the android pelvis is probably one of the most common variations of the pelvis which complicate obstetrics.

Robert pelvis   This pelvis has no wings (alae) of the sacrum and is therefore contracted in all diameters. It is a type very rarely seen and is the result of congenital abnormality. Caesarean section is always necessary for delivery.

Naegele pelvis   There is only one wing of the sacrum in this pelvis, giving it an obliquity. This may be due to congenital abnormality but can be caused by injury. A true Naegele pelvis is rarely seen, but some obliquity of the pelvis can also occur in a woman who has walked with a limp for many years. Delivery by caesarean section is always indicated.

THE PELVIC JOINTS IN PREGNANCY AND LABOUR

Towards the end of pregnancy there is an increase in the normal, minimal mobility of the pelvic joints. The alteration is brought about by the action of the hormone **relaxin** which acts on collagen, softening and causing relaxation of the pelvic ligaments. Relaxin is produced first by the corpus luteum and then by the developing placenta.

The symphysis pubis   Measured radiologically, the distance between the pubic bodies of a non-pregnant woman is on average 4 mm. In the last trimester of pregnancy this distance is widened by at least a further 3 mm, bringing about an increase in all pelvic diameters of brim, cavity and outlet. The fibrocartilaginous symphysis disc also softens and there is thinning and absorption of bone of the pubic bodies as well as the previously described changes which take place in the ligaments surrounding the joint.

In just a few women, the degree of symphysial widening is so great that when moving to a standing position, or when walking, there is movement of the pubic bodies. This condition is likely to cause pain as early as the 26th week of pregnancy and a firm corset needs to be worn for support.

During labour, in the presence of a minor degree of disproportion between the fetal head and pelvic brim, **symphysiotomy** might be carried out in remote areas of the world where full obstetric services are not available. The symphysis is widened surgically and delivery of the fetus is then usually facilitated by vacuum extraction. The widened joint is allowed to heal by the formation of fibrous tissue so that it is enlarged permanently and does not cause problems in subsequent pregnancies and labours. The 'operation' needs to be carried out by a person skilled in the procedure otherwise bladder trauma and orthopaedic complications can arise.

Hatfield (1973) reviewed the history and practice of this operation and estimated that for every 1 cm increase in joint width the capacity of the pelvis is increased by 8%.

Sacroiliac joints

Because these joints are well bound by strong ligaments they are normally capable of only very limited gliding and slight tilting movements. The latter movements are restrained by the sacro-tuberous and sacrospinous ligaments. Movement normally occurs only when:

1. Moving from a sitting to a standing position and vice versa
2. Lying on the back and raising an extended leg
3. Lying on the back and flexing the thighs – as for example in the lithotomy position.

At the period of pregnancy, when these pelvic joints are becoming more mobile and therefore less stable, they have to contend with the increasing weight of pregnancy being transmitted through the trunk and with the attitude of lordosis which so many women adopt towards the end of pregnancy. So it is not unusual in these last weeks for many women to complain of back pain and discomfort. The joints are being subjected to unaccustomed stress at a time when they are very vulnerable to it.

Sacrococcygeal joint

Allows the coccyx to continue its power of being able to tilt backwards and so facilitates passage of the fetal head during delivery.

Radiological investigation has demonstrated that, during uterine contractions and the descent of the fetal head through the pelvis, there is increased movement in all pelvic joints, together with a corresponding increase in pelvic capacity, as the diameters increase. The greatest variation occurs in primigravidae unless they are in the older age group.

The effect of the woman's position on pelvic capacity

Walcher's position

This is a very uncomfortable position for the pregnant woman to adopt. She lies on her back on a table or bed with her legs hyperextended over the edge.

In this position the ilium moves backwards and downwards at the sacroiliac joint, tilting the pelvis anteriorly. **This increases the diameter of the true conjugate at the pelvic brim – but there is a consequent reduction of available room at the outlet**.

This position favours descent of the fetal head into the pelvis and might perhaps be used in 'trial of labour'. But it is not very practical either from the view of comfort or of increasing the efficiency of uterine contractions. The position must of course be changed again to increase the capacity of the pelvic outlet. There is also some feeling that while this position does increase the measurements of the pelvic brim, the advantage is counteracted by the alteration of the angle of pelvic inclination at the brim.

Lithotomy With the woman lying on her back and with her hips and knees flexed, the pelvis is tilted posteriorly by movement at the sacroiliac joints. This has the opposite effect of Walcher's position. **The true conjugate of the pelvic brim is decreased in length, while the capacity of the outlet is increased**. It is therefore, in theory, a very suitable position for delivery of the fetal head in the second stage of labour. In practice many women dislike it because it is uncomfortable. Being 'strung up' they do not feel in control, neither can they see or assist their baby being born. It is also difficult to suckle a newly delivered infant when in the lithotomy position.

Nevertheless, the position has great value when, in the presence of a minor degree of pelvic outlet contraction, delivery is to be assisted with a forceps delivery or Ventouse extraction.

The lithotomy position can be modified by using a semi-recumbent position in which the mother flexes her thighs and knees. She may either pull up her own legs towards her during contractions or push her feet against an adaptation on the labour ward bed.

All fours or kneeling position Many women find this to be an uncomfortable position to maintain
(the lithotomy position for any length of time. As in the lithotomy position, **it reduces the**
turned upside down) **length of the true conjugate, but increases the capacity of the outlet**. The kneeling on all fours position is also of value in the first stage of labour when the occiput is presenting posteriorly. The position encourages the fetus to fall forwards and thus encourages rotation of the occiput to the anterior position.

Squatting In this position the thighs are abducted as well as flexed. The iliac crests move inwards as though the ilium were being squeezed together and the promontory of the sacrum moves downwards and forwards **reducing the true conjugate. The pubic angle is widened** because the ischial tuberosities move further apart; the coccyx moves upwards and backwards and **the outlet is enlarged** as the anteroposterior and transverse diameters are increased.

This squatting position for delivery of the infant has been an instinctive one in primitive societies over the centuries. Many women in our own society find it a natural one but it is probably used more as a modified knee squat position. Equipment used for monitoring the fetal heart or for intravenous or epidural therapy tends to hinder its use as does the fear of the infant being expelled too quickly and on to the floor. Some obstetric units have attempted to modify the 'squatting' position by using a 'birthing chair' or an adapted bed.

Effect of position on uterine action

Attwood (1976) demonstrated that uterine muscles exert most pressure when the labouring woman is in the sitting and squatting positions. Then, in decreasing order of pressure, he listed (1) standing, (2) semi-recumbent, (3) genupectoral kneeling, (4) recumbent.

POSTNATAL CONSIDERATIONS

The laxity of the pubic ligaments and increased mobility of the pelvic joints have great advantages during labour but their possible consequent effects need to be considered.

The **backache** and **discomfort** during pregnancy have been noted and these may continue into the postnatal period. Al Rawi & Al Rawi (1982) have suggested that changes which affect pelvic ligaments affect ligaments of the uterus equally and that such changes predispose to **prolapse of the uterus**.

Sacroiliac or sacrococcygeal strain caused during labour may also lead to back pain long after the puerperium is over. A supporting corset and physiotherapy may be required.

Advice should be given at the postnatal clinic if the mother is not already being treated by her GP.

REVISION QUESTIONS

Describe the bony pelvis. In your examination of the patient what might make you suspect the presence of a pelvic abnormality?

Describe the anatomy of the 'true' pelvis. What methods are adopted during pregnancy to ascertain that the pelvis is adequate for the passage of the child?

Describe the true pelvis. How may a narrow subpubic arch complicate labour?

Write short notes on:

1. The pelvic brim
2. Outlet of the bony pelvis
3. The true conjugate.

Describe the classification of pelves according to Caldwell and Molloy.

Describe the brim, cavity and outlet of the female pelvis. How may the pelvis be clinically assessed during the antenatal period?

Describe the bony pelvis. What is the obstetrical significance of the pelvic landmarks?

Describe the size, shape and landmarks of the gynaecoid pelvis. How would you use your knowledge of the pelvis in the management of labour?

How may variations in pelvic size and shape influence the outcome of labour?

Write short notes on:

1. The brim of the gynaecoid pelvis
2. Backache in pregnancy
3. Pelvic assessment
4. Delivery of the infant's shoulders
5. Anthropoid pelvis
6. Positions of a mother during labour and delivery
7. Ambulation during labour
8. The pelvic outlet
9. The importance of abdominal examination after 36th week of pregnancy.

REFERENCES AND FURTHER READING

Books and reports

Flint C 1986 Sensitive midwifery. Heinemann, London

Kapandji I A 1982 The physiology of the joints, 5th edn. Churchill Livingstone, Edinburgh

Mendez-Bauer C, Newton M 1983 Effects of different maternal positions during labour. Report of 5th European Congress on Perinatal Medicine, Uppsala. Perinatal Medicine (June): 208–211

Newton M 1986 Scientific foundations of obstetrics and gynaecology. Heinemann Medical, London

Articles

Al-Rawi Z S, Al-Rawi Z T 1982 Joint hypermobility in women with genital prolapse. Lancet i: 1439–1441

Armon P J, Philip M 1979 Symphysiotomy and subsequent pregnancy in the Kilimanjaro region of Tanzania. East African Medical Journal 55(7): 306–313

Attwood R J 1976 Parturitional posture and related birth behaviour. Acta Obstetricia et Gynaecologica Scandinavica (suppl) 57: 1–25

Biancuzzo M 1991 The patient observer: does the hands and knees position during labour help to rotate the OPP of the fetus? Birth 18(1): 40–43

Borrell U, Fernström I 1957 Movements at the sacro-iliac joint and their importance to changes in the pelvic dimensions during parturition. Acta Obstetricia et Gynaecologica Scandinavica 30: 36–42

Bryant-Greenwood G D 1985 Current concepts in the role of relaxin research in reproduction. IPPF (July)

Joseph J 1988 Joints of the pelvis and their relation to posture in labour. Midwives' Chronicle 101: 64

Mahmood T A, Campbell D M, Wilson A W 1988 Maternal height, shoe size and outcome of labour in white primigravidas: a prospective anthropomorphic study. British Medical Journal 297: 515–517

Palfrey A J 1974 The sex characteristics of the West African pelvis. MD thesis, University of Cambridge

Russell J G 1982 The rationale of primitive delivery positions. British Journal of Obstetrics and Gynaecology 89: 712–715

Stewart P, Spiby H 1988 Posture in labour. British Journal of Obstetrics and Gynaecology 96(1): 1258–1260

Stewart P et al 1983 A randomised trial to evaluate the use of a birth chair for delivery. Lancet i: 1296–1298

Stokes J 1987 The pelvic squeeze. Texas Midwifery 4(1): 10–11

3 The pelvic floor (or pelvic diaphragm)

(Plate 2B, Plate 3A and B, Plate 4A and B)

While the bony pelvis offers protection to the organs it encloses, it can by no means support them unaided. However, the pelvis and the ligaments make a framework where muscles can originate and insert (Fig. 3.1). Muscles and ligaments providing the framework are:

- *Sacrospinous ligament*
- *Sacrotuberous ligament*   extend across the greater and lesser
- *Piriformis muscle*   sciatic notches
- *Gluteus maximus muscle*
- *Obturator internus muscle*: stretches across the obturator foramen
- *White line of fascia*: a condensation of the obturator internus muscle (arcus tendineus fasciae) which extends from each ischial spine to the same pubic body. It is an area on the lateral pelvic walls where the deep pelvic muscles originate.

The outlet of the bony pelvis is filled with soft tissues which support the pelvic and abdominal organs. These tissues form not a flat floor but a gutter-shaped structure which is higher posteriorly

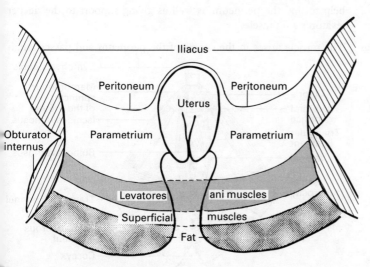

Fig. 3.1 Tissue layers of pelvic floor.

Iliacus
Peritoneum
Uterus
Peritoneum
Obturator internus
Parametrium
Parametrium
Levatores ani muscles
Superficial muscles
Fat

47

than anteriorly. Three canals, each with an external orifice, run through the tissues: the urethra, the vagina and the rectum. There are six layers of tissue:

1. An outer covering of *skin*
2. *Subcutaneous fat*
3. *Superficial muscles* enclosed in fascia
4. *Deep muscles* enclosed in fascia
5. *Pelvic fascia* thickened to form *pelvic ligaments*
6. *Peritoneum.*

SUPERFICIAL PELVIC FLOOR MUSCLES
(Fig. 3.2)

These muscles are of less importance than the levatores ani muscles which lie above them but they provide additional strength to the deep musculature by their support.

They include:

- *Transversus perinei muscle*
- *Bulbocavernosus muscle*
- *Ischiocavernosus muscle*
- *External anal sphincter*
- Muscles which control the *external urinary meatus*
- The *triangular ligaments* } fill the remaining spaces
- The *ischiorectal fat*

Transversus perinei   One muscle arises from the inner surface of each ischial tuberosity and passes transversely across the outlet to meet its fellow. Fibres of each muscle unite and intermingle in the superficial tissues of the perineal body. Some fibres continue posteriorly and blend with fibres of the external anal sphincter. The transverse perinei muscles help to 'fix' the perineum as well as giving support to the deeper levatores ani muscle.

Bulbocavernosus   The muscle arises in the centre of the perineum and passes longi-

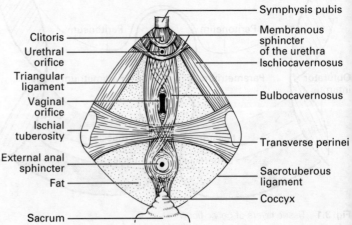

Clitoris —
Urethral orifice —
Triangular ligament —
Vaginal orifice —
Ischial tuberosity —
External anal sphincter —
Fat —
Sacrum —

Symphysis pubis
Membranous sphincter of the urethra
Ischiocavernosus
Bulbocavernosus
Transverse perinei
Sacrotuberous ligament
Coccyx

Fig. 3.2 Superficial muscles of pelvic floor.

tudinal fibres on each side of the urethra and vagina, encircling both orifices before inserting into the corpus of the clitoris. These anterior fibres allow erection of the clitoris during sexual activity. Where the urethra pierces the pelvic floor, muscle fibres compress the lumen of its distal portion to form the compressor urethrae or membranous sphincter of the urethra. The muscle fibres surrounding the vagina aid contraction of the vaginal walls during intercourse.

Like the transverse perinei, this muscle also supports the levator ani muscle which lies deeper to it.

Ischiocavernosus   One muscle runs from each ischial tuberosity to the clitoris and the fibres interweave with those composing the membranous sphincter of the urethra. The fascia of these muscles helps to fill the anterior space of the pelvic outlet.

External anal sphincter   is a ring of muscle surrounding the anus. It is formed by the merging of muscle fibres from the superficial and deep layers. The fourchette and perineal skin partly cover the sphincter.

External urinary meatus   is the opening of the distal portion of the urethra which is compressed by muscle fibres. This 'sphincter' is analogous to the male sphincter which has the same name, but in the female it is a weaker and less important structure. The orifice has an everted edge which sometimes makes it difficult to find when wanting to pass a urinary catheter. It must be differentiated from the clitoris, which should be identified first.

The outlet of the pelvis still has four areas which need to be filled with tissue if it is to be supportive. These are filled by the triangular ligaments and ischiorectal fat.

Triangular ligaments   Two triangular areas lie anteriorly and are bounded by the ischiocavernosus and transverse perinei muscles. They are filled with musculomembranous tissue and have inferior and superior layers of fascia, extensions from the fascia of the ischiocavernosus muscles. As well as completing the unfilled area of the pelvic outlet, these 'ligaments' give additional support to the neck of the bladder because they stretch right across the pubic arch.

Ischiorectal fossa   This is bounded by the gluteus maximus muscle, overlaid by the sacrospinous ligament at one side and by the transverse perinei and bulbocavernosus muscles on the other. This area is filled with fat.

Blood supply   Blood supply is through branches of the internal iliac artery and veins.

Lymphatic drainage   Lymphatic drainage is into the inguinal glands.

Nerve supply   Nerve supply is from the 3rd and 4th segments of the sacral plexus and the pudendal nerve.

DEEP PELVIC FLOOR MUSCLES (Fig. 3.3)

These lie at a deeper level in the pelvis and above the superficial

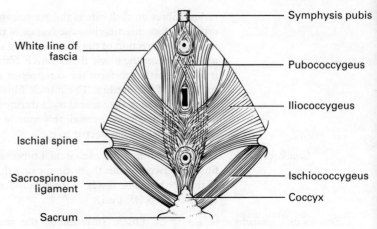

White line of fascia — Symphysis pubis — Pubococcygeus — Iliococcygeus — Ischial spine — Sacrospinous ligament — Ischiococcygeus — Coccyx — Sacrum

Fig. 3.3 Deep muscles of pelvic floor (levatores ani muscles).

layer. They are about 5 mm in depth. They each have their insertion around the coccyx and are therefore sometimes called the coccygeal muscles. These muscles, although aided by the superficial layer, are of vital importance in the voluntary control of the bladder and bowels. The hygiene, comfort and social wellbeing of a woman, as well as her childbearing ability, are therefore dependent upon the effectiveness of their muscle tone. There are three pairs of muscles which make up each levator ani muscle:

Iliococcygeus arises from the white line of fascia on the inner aspect of each iliac bone and from each ischial spine and runs posteriorly to the coccyx. Fibres from the right and left sides meet midline in front of the coccyx and join with other fibres to form the superficial layer, namely the anal sphincter and transverse perinei muscles.

Ischiococcygeus arises from each ischial spine and passes to the upper part of the coccyx and lower border of the sacrum. Posteriorly then, the pelvic diaphragm is now almost closed. These muscles help to stabilise the sacroiliac and sacrococcygeal joints.

Pubococcygeus Each muscle arises from the inner border of the body of the pubic bone and from the white line of fascia. They then sweep posteriorly in three distinct bands. A central band of fibres surrounds the urethra. Some make a U-loop around the vagina and insert into the lateral and posterior vaginal wall and into the central part of the perineum. Some fibres continue posteriorly and form a loop around the anus, inserting into the lateral and posterior walls of the anal canal. They insert finally into the coccyx.

The pubococcygeus muscles are the most important of all the pelvic floor muscles. They surround and support the urethra, vagina and rectum. Controlled micturition and defaecation, as well as normal sexual function, are dependent upon them.

Blood supply Blood supply is from the pudendal arteries, branches of the internal iliac artery. Venous drainage is into corresponding veins.

Lymphatic drainage Lymphatic drainage is into the inguinal and external iliac glands.

Nerve supply   Nerve supply is from the 3rd and 4th sacral nerves. The 5th sacral nerve and the coccygeal nerve pass through but do not serve these muscles.

THE PERINEAL BODY (Fig. 3.4)

Situation   It lies between the vaginal and rectal canals.

Shape   It is triangular, the base being the skin and the apex pointing upwards.

Size   Each side of the triangle is approximately 3.5 cm in length.

Structure   There are three layers of tissue:

1. Outer covering of skin
2. *Superficial pelvic floor muscles*
   a. Bulbocavernosus
   b. Transverse perinei
3. *Deep pelvic floor muscle* – pubococcygeus.

Blood supply   The blood supply is from the pudendal arteries, branches of the internal iliac artery. Venous drainage is into the corresponding veins.

Lymphatic drainage   Lymphatic drainage is into the inguinal and external iliac glands.

Nerve supply   Nerve supply is from the perineal branch of the pudendal nerve.

Function   The function of the perineal body is to assist in the process of defaecation and childbirth. During the latter function, the structure may become overstretched or torn, and the midwife must learn how

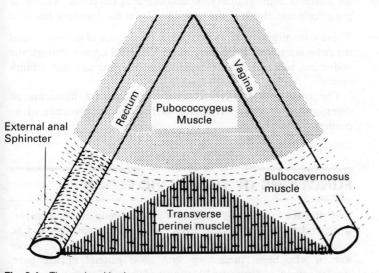

Fig. 3.4   The perineal body.

such injuries can be minimised. Trauma may result in disorders of micturition and bowel function and in prolapse of the pelvic, and sometimes even of the abdominal, organs.

PELVIC FASCIA

Pelvic fascia is a combination of connective tissue, blood vessels and voluntary and involuntary muscle fibres. It lines the walls and floor of the pelvic cavity and fills the areas between the organs, thus giving additional support but still allowing each organ to move within the limits of normal function. In areas where organs need extra support the fascia thickens to form pelvic ligaments. These are:

Two lateral ligaments   extend from the white line of fascia to the lateral walls of the bladder.

Two pubovesical ligaments   extend from the neck of the bladder to the inner surface of each pubic body. They form part of the pubocervical ligaments.

These ligaments are supports of the bladder

Two pubocervical ligaments   are attached to the inner surface of each pubic body; they run posteriorly and become attached to the neck of the bladder, the vault of the vagina and the supravaginal cervix.

These ligaments support the bladder and the uterus

Transverse cervical ligaments   (also known as the *cardinal or Mackenrodt's* ligaments) are attached to the vaginal vault and supravaginal cervix. They run transversely across the pelvic floor and fan out until they reach the white line of fascia. They are the strongest of the pelvic ligaments.

Uterosacral ligaments   are attached to the vaginal vault and supravaginal cervix. They pass posteriorly and attach to the lateral border of the 1st sacral body.

Round ligaments   These arise anteriorly from just below the cornua of the uterus and the fallopian tubes. They then take a V-shaped course through the abdominal wall and inguinal canal before inserting into each labium majus.

The transverse cervical, uterosacral and round ligaments all contribute to the support of the uterus and maintenance of its position.

FUNCTIONS OF THE PELVIC FLOOR

The effective functioning of the pelvic floor (the pelvic diaphragm) is dependent upon the maintenance of good muscle tone and an equality of balanced muscle on each side of the pelvis. Those women who begin pregnancy with good general muscle tone, regular activity and exercise being part of their daily routine, are less

likely to suffer pelvic floor trauma during childbirth than those women who lead sedentary lives. Its healthy functioning is imperative
if micturition and defaecation are to be controlled and normal
sexual activity is to be enjoyed by women of all ages.

Support   The pubococcygeus muscle is a most important structure of
support since it surrounds the urethral, vaginal and rectal orifices.
Its principal function is to support the vagina (which helps to
support the uterus), as well as the bladder, urethra and rectum. It is
also the muscle which is most vulnerable during childbirth. Nevertheless all muscles offer support, the superficial muscles reinforcing
the deep layer.

Maintenance of   Activities such as laughing, sneezing, coughing, vomiting, as well as
intra-abdominal   micturition, defaecation and labour contractions, all cause a rise in
pressure   intra-abdominal pressure. The muscles of the pelvic floor therefore
need to be in a constant state of tone and respond reflexly if they are
to hold the pelvic organs in position.

Relaxation   The hormone **relaxin** effects relaxation of the pelvic floor muscles
and ligaments during pregnancy, softens them and prepares for the
distension of tissues which takes place in the second stage of labour.
This softening of tissues makes the performance of vaginal
examination much easier towards the end of pregnancy and in
labour and causes less discomfort to the woman.

Expulsive action in   During defaecation, the diaphragm, abdominal muscles and pelvic
defaecation and   floor muscles are all contracted. Faeces are propelled into the anus,
childbirth   causing relaxation of the deep muscles supporting the rectal wall.
The superficial muscles are pulled upwards over the faecal mass
and then there is a 'bearing down' expulsive movement. Similarly,
in labour, the fetus passes through the vagina, but an enormous
distension of the walls is needed. This is possible because laterally,
the fat in the ischiorectal fossae can be temporarily compressed
while the fetus is passing through. Anteriorly, the bladder should be
empty and is drawn up into the abdomen because of its attachment
to the lower uterine segment. (The urethra becomes elongated.)
Posteriorly, the rectum and posterior part of the pelvic floor are
pushed downwards and backward and simultaneously the anterior
part of the pelvic floor is pulled upwards and forwards. The perineum stretches and bulges visibly, the rectum is flattened and its
anterior wall can be seen as the anus undergoes extreme dilatation.
This displacement increases the length of the vaginal walls, which
follow the same curve as the canal of the bony pelvis. Expulsion of
the fetus is aided by maternal effort in 'bearing down' movements.
At the completion of labour, pelvic floor tissues return to their
normal position but muscles will need to regain their tone.

PERINEAL TRAUMA

Stretching of muscles   Even if no lacerations have occurred, it should be borne in mind that all the tissues of the perineum have been subjected to compression during the second stage of labour as well as being dilated or elongated.

Minor laceration   of the labia or grazes of the perineal skin. Such lacerations are painful but not serious.

First degree tear   is a minor laceration which involves only the fourchette and perineal skin.

Second degree tear   The skin, mucous membrane and superficial pelvic floor muscles are involved and will quite possibly be accompanied by lacerations of the labia and/or vaginal walls. If the tear is deep, the levatores ani muscles are involved.

Third degree tear   This is much more serious because not only are the deep muscles involved but the tear extends so far posteriorly that the anterior area of the external anal sphincter is involved.

Fourth degree tear   The tear extends into the anterior wall of the rectum to involve the internal sphincter of the anus. (This classification is of wider use in America than in the UK.)

Third and fourth degree perineal tears should be sutured as soon as possible after delivery by a skilled obstetrician. If not treated skilfully, they can result in faecal and flatus incontinence. Whether or not perineal lacerations occur during labour, it should be borne in mind that the soft tissues and the nerves supplying them have all been subject to tremendous pressure and gross distension as the fetus passes through the birth canal. Electrophysiological diagnostic techniques can now be used to demonstrate that the pudendal nerve which supplies both the pubococcygeus muscle and the external sphincter of the urethra and anus, is commonly damaged during childbirth. A lax pubococcygeus muscle will also alter the angle of the urethrovesical and anorectal junction, contributing to incontinence or stress incontinence of urine and/or faeces (see Ch. 4). The damage is largely related to the second stage of labour and there is a higher incidence associated with multiparity and instrumental delivery. Conversely, in elective caesarean section when the fetus is not expelled through the pelvic canal, there is no associated pelvic floor denervation. The long-term effects of pelvic floor trauma are listed at the end of this chapter.

PREVENTION OF PELVIC FLOOR TRAUMA

Antenatal period

It is of prime importance that wherever her delivery is to take place – in a specialist obstetric unit, GP unit, at home or elsewhere – the pregnant woman should feel entirely content that it is a 'safe' place. From the time of her very first visit to her obstetrician, GP or midwife she needs the assurance of being in caring and competent hands. She should be encouraged to express her own opinions about the conduct of her pregnancy and labour both with the midwife and at educational sessions with other pregnant women and their husbands. This is often difficult in a large obstetric unit but it is an ideal to be aimed at. A confident and relaxed woman who feels at home in her labour ward situation, who has been adequately prepared for this birth day, is much more likely to be in control when labour actually commences. She is also much more likely to accept any guidance about her delivery that the midwife feels is advisable.

During the antenatal period, the following points are especially relevant to the prevention of perineal trauma:

General health, including prevention or treatment of anaemia. A healthy body with tissues which are nourished with a good blood supply will always function more satisfactorily than one which is undernourished and not kept in good form.

Exercise Any form of exercise which improves muscle tone should be encouraged, providing that it is neither dangerous nor too strenuous.

Walking, swimming, dancing, cycling, riding can all be safely continued for as long as the woman feels able. Those who do not commence pregnancy with a 'keep-fit' orientation might be encouraged to take up some gentle forms of exercise such as walking rather than driving or using public transport. There is still considerable controversy as to the value of antenatal exercises – some believe that pregnancy is too late to start trying to improve muscle tone. Students should make themselves aware of their own hospital policy but keep an open mind. Perineal 'awareness' should certainly be taught and, as well as contracting and relaxing these muscles regularly, the mother should be encouraged to stretch her perineum as much as possible by squatting and sitting cross legged on the floor for as long as pregnancy allows. Oiling and massaging of the perineum is currently believed to be beneficial in making the tissues more supple.

Assessment of pelvic floor tone While the mother is lying on the examination couch at the first antenatal visit, she should be asked by the obstetrician to 'bear down' as in defaecation. Bulging of the perineum will indicate poor pelvic floor muscle tone and may be accompanied by stress urinary or faecal incontinence. In this event some obstetricians will elect to deliver this woman by caesarean section. Similarly, a woman who has already undergone pelvic floor repair would not usually be considered as suitable for vaginal delivery.

Discussion The mother should be encouraged to express her own ideas about the management of her labour and who she would like to be with her. There should be mutual discussion with the midwife concerning the alternatives of episiotomy or the allowing of a perineal tear, the advantages or disadvantages of the various delivery positions and any other subjects which might be of concern to her.

Health education   A basic knowledge of the process of labour should be taught or revised and the mother should be shown how she can carry out special breathing techniques in the first and second stages. The use of inhalational analgesia can be demonstrated and the technique for breathing out the baby's head practised.

During labour

First stage   Ideally, the woman should not be admitted to a labour ward until she is in established labour. General activity should be encouraged until that time. Basic nursing management relating to her position, comfort and relaxation, ambulation if she wishes, companionship and occupation, light diet, warm baths are all important factors in the first stage of labour and are described fully in most midwifery textbooks. The subject of positions in labour was introduced in Chapter 2.

Special points to bear in mind during the first stage of labour, in the prevention of pelvic floor trauma, include:

1. A reminder, each hour during the first stage, that the bladder should be emptied.
2. If the woman has a strong urge to 'bear down' before the cervix is fully dilated, then the foot of the bed should be raised if she is in bed, and analgesia is advisable. Alternatively, she may be encouraged to lie on her side or to adopt a kneeling position with her chest and abdomen supported. These positions relieve the pressure of the fetal head on the cervix and rectum. The administration of inhalational analgesia at the time of contractions will also be helpful to her (see Ch. 8, p. 124).

'Bearing down' before the cervix is fully dilated results in oedema of the cervix and prolongation of the first stage, as well as causing overstretching of pelvic floor muscles and pelvic ligaments.

Second stage

Position   Some research has been carried out regarding the effect on the perineal muscles when the fetus is expelled through the birth canal. Kneeling, squatting and modified sitting positions are instinctive in primitive peoples, leading us to suppose that this not only aids expulsion of the fetus but minimises the pain and therefore possibly the trauma associated with perineal stretching.

In the UK the left lateral position (with the mother's upper leg raised) was once very commonly used. It was taught that this resulted in fewer perineal tears but there is little evidence to support this.

Skilful delivery   In the second stage of labour (the stage of expulsion of the fetus) careful attention must be paid to delivery of the fetal head. The mother should be asked to 'breathe' out the fetal head between contractions. The smallest possible diameters of the fetal skull must be allowed to distend the vulva and perineum. This is a technique which can only be learned by practical experience during midwifery practice. The midwife must keep her hands off the perineum. Handling is likely to cause bruising of these greatly distended tissues and bruised tissues tear more easily.

If there is a delay in the descent of the fetal head, then an obstetrician should be informed. The wise use of episiotomy (surgical incision of the perineum) and forceps delivery will prevent excessive trauma to both the perineum and the fetal head.

Once the head has been delivered, the midwife must wait for the anterior shoulder to rotate and come to lie under the pubic arch. The large diameter of the shoulders is then lying in the anteroposterior diameter of the pelvic outlet where most room is available. The anterior shoulder should then be allowed to escape, after which the baby's body is taken upwards in a movement of lateral flexion over the mother's abdomen. This allows the posterior shoulder and the baby to escape through the curved birth canal without further pressure on the perineum.

A midwife who has gained the confidence and trust of the woman throughout pregnancy is more likely to find her co-operative and in control during the second stage of labour, thus further minimising trauma. Therefore, wherever possible, antenatal mothers should have the opportunity of meeting the midwives who are likely to be on duty in the labour ward. At such a meeting there can be a visit to the labour ward, an informal discussion about any positions they wish to adopt for delivery and any special needs that the mother is concerned about.

Postnatally

While specific pelvic floor exercises are of some value in restoring pelvic floor muscle tone, even greater benefit is obtained by general exercise and the mother should be encouraged to resume normal physical activities and exercise as soon as possible.

EPISIOTOMY

Definition Episiotomy is a surgical incision of the perineum which is carried out prior to the delivery of the infant.

There is now considerable discussion as to whether an episiotomy really is preferable to a perineal tear.

Those in favour of episiotomy believe that:

1. It prevents extensive perineal trauma and protects the anal sphincter muscles
2. It reduces compression of the fetal skull
3. It heals more neatly
4. In the long term is prevents postnatal laxity of the pelvic floor muscles.

The alternative view is that:

1. An episiotomy wound has a higher incidence of breakdown than a sutured spontaneous laceration
2. An episiotomy suture line causes more pain to the mother than a sutured spontaneous laceration
3. Even when healed, the episiotomy causes a wider introitus and defective perineal tissues
4. The long term result of 3. predisposes to:
   a. vaginal infection
   b. an impairment of sexual response sometimes to the degree of dyspareunia.

There is a general belief now, however, that an episiotomy should not be a routine procedure but should be carried out only for a specific purpose.

Indications

To expedite delivery   in the following circumstances:

- Pre-eclampsia
- Eclampsia (if labour is too advanced for caesarean section to be carried out)
- Cardiac or respiratory disease ⎫
- Previous pelvic floor repair   ⎬ if vaginal delivery is elected
- Maternal distress   ⎭
- Fetal distress
- Cord prolapse (if mother is in the second stage of labour and delivery is imminent)
- Prior to forceps delivery or ventouse extraction.

To prevent excessive trauma:
1. Rigid perineum
2. Buttonholing of perineum
3. Previous third degree tear
4. Presence of female circumcision scarring
5. Prior to forceps delivery
6. Persistent occipitoposterior delivery
7. Face delivery
8. Narrow pubic arch.

To prevent cerebral damage:
1. Slow advance of fetal head
2. Prematurity
3. Aftercoming head of the breech.

TECHNIQUE

Preparation of the mother   If the midwife believes that an episiotomy really is necessary, then she should suggest this fact to the woman in labour and to her husband, if he is present. Without causing anxiety to them, she should explain why she believes it to be needful and gain their assent. An explanation of episiotomy will, one hopes, have been given at antenatal classes since it is unlikely that there would, at that stage, be time for teaching and long explanations. However, a reminder that she will have a local anaesthetic and then her tissues widened so that the baby can be delivered more easily should at least be given. Because there is a possibility that any person may suffer a drug reaction, the mother should also be asked if she has ever previously had a local anaesthetic and whether or not there was an adverse reaction. In sensitive people, reaction is shown by a fall in blood pressure, respiration which becomes distressed and then convulsions.

Infiltration of the perineum

Episiotomy should be regarded as an aseptic procedure and the surrounding skin area should be cleansed.

10 ml of lignocaine 0.5% is drawn up into a syringe and an intramuscular needle is then attached. Air bubbles must be excluded.

The needle is inserted into the fourchette at the midline and passes subcutaneously into the perineal skin along the chosen site for episiotomy for a distance of 4 cm, and a little lignocaine is infiltrated. (The piston should be withdrawn before the injection to ensure that no blood vessels have been penetrated.) Having made sure that all is well, 3 ml of lignocaine is then injected as the needle is slowly withdrawn, thus ensuring that it does not enter a vein. The needle is then withdrawn almost completely and its direction is changed, first to the right and then the left of the original injection, 3 ml of lignocaine being infiltrated on each side. A fan-shaped area is thus anaesthetised.

Those midwives who have suffered at the hands of an overworked dentist will know only too well that a full 5 minutes need to elapse before full loss of sensation is achieved. The woman in labour also requires that 5 minutes for a local anaesthetic to take effect!

Types of episiotomy (Fig. 3.5)

There is current controversy not only about the use of episiotomy but also about the direction in which the incision should be made. The student must be aware of the policy within her own unit.

The medial incision

This, and every other type of incision here described, is made with long, blunt-ended scissors. The medial incision is made in the midline from the centre of the fourchette, is about 2.5 cm in length and passes posteriorly towards the anus. When this central incision is made the muscles involved are:

1. *The transverse perinei muscles*, whose fibres run transversely between the centre of the perineum and each ischial tuberosity. Their fibres interlace centrally in the perineum.
2. *The bulbocavernosus muscles*: these fibres run longitudinally from the point where they arise in the centre of the perineum. Some of them surround the vaginal orifice.
3. *The pubococcygeus muscles*: Some fibres pass longitudinally from the pubic bodies and insert into the lateral and posterior vaginal walls and into the centre of the perineum.

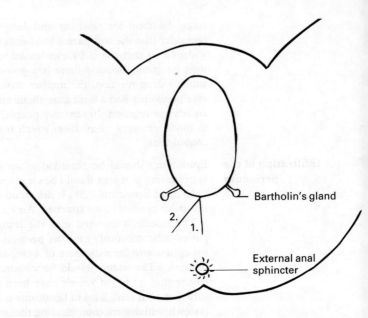

Bartholin's gland

2. 1.

External anal
sphincter

Fig. 3.5 Types of
episiotomy: (1) medial
(2) mediolateral.

4. *The iliococcygeus muscles*: Fibres from the right and left muscles
meet in the midline to join and interlace with fibres from the
above-mentioned muscles.

This incision increases the anteroposterior diameter of the outlet
of the pelvic floor. Because these muscles all meet centrally, a
medial incision will not affect muscle balance of the right and left
sides of the pelvic floor and they will be easy to repair as they can be
easily aligned. There are fewer blood vessels in this central area and
bleeding is therefore minimal. Postnatally there is little discomfort
while healing takes place and, in the long term, dyspareunia is rare.

Disadvantages The disadvantage most commonly expressed is that the incision is
more likely to extend to involve the anus. There is no general agree-
ment on this and some obstetric units have proved it not to be true
(Beynon 1974).

Nevertheless, if the woman has had a previous third degree tear, a
skilled obstetrician might prefer to perform the episiotomy himself.
If the woman has a short perineum with less than 4 cm between the
vaginal orifice and the anus, there is also a greater risk that the
external sphincter and posterior rectal wall could be lacerated.

**The mediolateral
incision**

This incision is also commenced in the midline at the centre of the
fourchette, then runs posteriorly midway between the ischial spine
and the anus. Some midwives and obstetricians choose this incision
if the woman has a short perineum, has had a previous third degree
tear or if large diameters of the fetal head (e.g. persistent occipito
posterior position) are presenting.

Disadvantages By making a lateral incision the equal balance of the pelvic floor is
distorted and the muscles are less easy to align and suture. If the

incision extends upwards then it could extend into the cervix. The area incised is rich in venous plexuses and the wound may bleed heavily.

Postnatally the wound breaks down more often than a medial suture line and there is a certain amount of healing by secondary intention. An unsightly and tender scar is the result. In the long term it leaves a wider introitus and defective perineal muscles.

J-shaped incision As its name implies, the incision commences as a medial episiotomy and then turns outwards to avoid the anus. The only advantage of this incision is that the external anal sphincter is avoided.

Disadvantages It is very difficult to suture and has all the disadvantages of the mediolateral incision.

To make the incision

Two fingers are placed in the vagina, as for infiltration of the perineum, and are used as before to distinguish the area and to protect the fetal head.

The incision is started in the midline and is directed along the chosen line of incision. It is made through the perineal skin and muscles with one determined cut approximately 4 cm in length. The incision should be made during a uterine contraction when the perineal tissues are thinned, so that bleeding is controlled by pressure of the fetal head.

REPAIR OF EPISIOTOMY

Since 1970, midwives who have been trained in the technique of perineal repair are now permitted to suture a perineal tear or episiotomy, unsupervised, in most instances. As far as possible, the midwife who performed the episiotomy should also suture it and the repair should be carried out promptly. Physically, this is more conducive to healing and there is less risk of wound infection and subsequent breakdown.

Emotionally, too, this is far more satisfactory for the newly delivered mother who, after the climax of delivering her baby, wants to be bathed and left alone to enjoy him. The days of prolonged waiting for perineal suturing should not be suffered today by the majority of newly-delivered mothers.

Most obstetricians will issue guidelines concerning when it is advisable for medical aid to be sought prior to suturing, and such conditions will include:

- An extended episiotomy or third degree tear
- Perineal tear or episiotomy with vaginal wall lacerations
- History of previous third degree tear
- Presence of existing extensive scarring of perineum or scarring resulting from female circumcision
- Varicose veins of the vulva.

Where there has been a forceps delivery or ventouse extraction, an obstetrician will be present and will usually repair the episiotomy himself.

Preparation for suturing   Strict aseptic technique should be observed.

It is important to explain to the mother why suturing is required. Her husband should be allowed to stay if they both wish it. Talk to the mother and tell her what you are doing as you do it and continue to talk as suturing is taking place. She is no doubt anxious and feeling that this is an anticlimax. The mother's general condition should be assessed and it should be ascertained that the uterus is well contracted.

Prior to preparation of the patient, the placenta and membranes should be inspected to ensure that there are no retained products. To discover this *after* the perineum has been sutured is a crime of negligence.

A good Anglepoise®-type light is essential; it should be directed on to the perineum.

Anaesthetic prior to suturing   If the mother has had an epidural or pudendal block, or has been given a local anaesthetic prior to episiotomy, it is unlikely that further anaesthesia will be required if suturing is carried out immediately following completion of the third stage and examination of the placenta and membranes.

Should it be required, 10 ml of lignocaine 1% may be given within one hour of that given for episiotomy, or the use of entonox may be adequate. The standard hospital procedure should be followed here, as it should for suturing the perineum, but the main points to bear in mind include:

1. *Cleansing before suturing*: Blood clots should be removed from the vagina and any bleeding vessels should be clamped until they can be ligated. It is useful to place a taped tampon high into the vagina so that blood does not obscure the lacerated tissues. The tampon must be recorded and included in the swab count and it must be removed at the end of the procedure
2. *Vaginal walls* are usually sutured *first*
3. *Muscles* of the perineal body are sutured *next*
4. The *skin is closed*
5. The *tampon is removed* and included in the swab count.

DISADVANTAGES OF EPISIOTOMY

1. It is a mutilation if used without very good cause
2. The scar may cause dyspareunia if sutured too tightly
3. If the wound is not sutured tightly enough, the vagina is lax and there is less pleasurable sensation for both partners in sexual intercourse
4. Resultant scar tissue may make episiotomy necessary at subsequent deliveries.

CARE FOLLOWING DELIVERY

Lacerations will heal more readily and tissues regain their tone more readily if the following points are observed:

1. Lacerations must be sutured promptly
2. The wound must be kept as clean and dry as possible
3. Gentle and graduated pelvic floor exercises should be taught
4. Ambulation should be encouraged
5. Attention must be paid to general health
6. Anaemia should be prevented or treated
7. Non-absorbent sutures should be removed alternately on sixth and seventh days.

During the early postnatal period, perineal pain can be relieved by local applications such as ice packs or witch-hazel compresses. The oral administration of a drug containing proteolytic enzymes is sometimes beneficial because the drug reduces inflammation and oedema by acting on the soft fibrin deposits in the tissues. Applications of witch-hazel have the same effect but need to be used almost immediately after suturing. The mother should be encouraged to wash the suture line gently with a soaped hand and massage movements when she is in the bath or using the bidet and then to dry the area with absorbent tissues. Massage encourages circulation and aids the healing processes.

Should perineal pain persist while the mother is in hospital, then the physiotherapist may be consulted concerning the use of ultrasound or infrared treatment.

This type of pain will indirectly affect breast feeding. The mother will therefore most probably need assistance in finding a comfortable position in which to feed her baby.

POSTNATAL EXAMINATION

In addition to monitoring the general wellbeing of the mother, a vaginal examination is carried out at this examination, 6 weeks after delivery.

This is to assess:

1. That all vaginal, cervical and perineal lacerations have healed
2. The tone of the pelvic floor muscles by asking the patient to 'bear down' or cough. The muscles should not bulge downwards
3. In conjunction with 2. to diagnose any degree of urinary incontinence, faecal or flatus incontinence
4. That sexual intercourse has been resumed satisfactorily.

Where any effects of trauma are evident, the postnatal mother is referred to the physiotherapy department and possibly the gynaecological department for treatment.

LONG-TERM EFFECTS OF UNTREATED PELVIC FLOOR TRAUMA

- Stress incontinence of urine
- Incontinence of urine
- Stress incontinence of faeces
- Dyspareunia
- Cystocele
- Urethrocele
- Rectocele
- Uterine prolapse
- Complete procidentia
- Retroverted uterus.

In 1983 the National Childbirth Trust carried out a survey to try to establish whether or not episiotomy reduced the incidence of prolapse of the uterus. Only 728 women out of 3000 answered the survey but of those who replied, the majority had had normal deliveries. The survey was followed up in 1985 and the organisers were surprised to discover that one-half of those who replied suffered from symptoms associated with damage to pelvic floor muscles, i.e. dyspareunia and increased frequency of micturition, while 37% complained of stress incontinence.

No simple relationship between episiotomy and the incidence of uterine prolapse was discovered, but what gave cause for concern was the number of women who accepted ongoing stress incontinence as an inevitable consequence of childbirth. Midwives must be aware of their responsibility for health education in this respect.

REVISION QUESTIONS

What are the causes of lacerations of the perineum during delivery? Describe how you would attempt to avoid a perineal tear during a normal vertex delivery.

Describe the vagina and perineum. How may injuries to these structures be minimised during labour and delivery?

Describe the perineal body. How may this be damaged in labour and what steps can be taken to minimise this danger?

What are the indications for episiotomy? When should a midwife undertake this procedure? Describe the technique she might employ.

What anatomical structures are incised during the procedure of episiotomy? What are the advantages and disadvantages of this procedure?

Describe the anatomy of the perineal body. Explain in detail how the midwife would repair an episiotomy.

Describe in detail how the midwife would perform an episiotomy. What are the advantages of a midwife undertaking perineal repair? Discuss postnatal care of the wound.

What are the indications for episiotomy? Describe in detail how an episiotomy should be carried out. What anatomical structures will be incised during the procedure? Discuss the care of the wound during the immediate postnatal period.

Pelvic floor damage may impair a woman's health. Describe the anatomy of the pelvic floor. How may the midwife prevent or minimise pelvic floor damage?

Describe the perineal body. Discuss the effects on a woman of perineal discomfort in the puerperium. How will the midwife manage the situation?

Describe the anatomy of the pelvic floor. What are the causes of a third degree tear? How may the midwife reduce the risk of such a tear?

Describe the anatomy of the perineal body. Outline the ways in which the midwife may prevent or minimise

1. damage to the pelvic floor in labour
2. perineal pain during the early postnatal period.

Write short notes on:

- Care of a sutured perineum
- Difficulties with sexual intercourse when the woman has had a perineal repair
- Alleviation of perineal discomfort 6 weeks after delivery
- Perineal pain in the postnatal period
- Effect on a woman of perineal suturing
- Shoulder dystocia
- Indications for performing an episiotomy
- Prevention of perineal damage
- Recognition of perineal problems in the postnatal period.

REFERENCES AND FURTHER READING

Books and reports
Chard T, Richard M 1977 Benefits and hazards of the new obstetrics. Heinemann, London
Kitzinger S 1984 The experience of childbirth. Penguin, Harmondsworth
Kitzinger S 1984 Episiotomy and the second stage of labour. Penny Press, ?
Polden M, Mantle J 1990 Physiotherapy in obstetrics and gynaecology. Butterworth-Heinemann, London
Whiteford B, Polden M 1988 Postnatal exercises: a six-month fitness programme for mother and baby. Century, London

Articles
Avery M D, Van Arsdale L 1987 Perineal massage: effect on the incidence of episiotomy and laceration in a nulliparous population. Journal of Nursing and Midwifery 32(3): 181–184
Baker G 1981 The unkindest cut of all? World Medicine (Aug 8): 40–41
Banter D, Thacker S 1982 Risks and benefit of episiotomy. Birth 9: 25–30
Beischer N 1967 The anatomical and functional results of medio-lateral episiotomy. Midwifery Times of Australia 2: 189
Beynon C L 1974 Midline episiotomy as a routine procedure. Journal of Obstetrics and Gynaecology of the British Commonwealth 81: 126
Cronk M 1987 Perineal suturing. Nursing Times (Feb): 62

Dougherty M 1989 The effect of exercise on the circumvaginal muscles in post-partum women. Journal of Nursing and Midwifery 34(1): 8–13

Fleming N 1990 Can the suturing method make a difference in post-partum perineal pain. Journal of Nursing and Midwifery 35(1): 19–25

Gordon H, Cogue M 1985 Perineal muscle function after childbirth. Lancet 2: 123–125

Grant A 1986 Repair of episiotomies and perineal tears. British Journal of Obstetrics and Gynaecology 93(5): 417–419

Greenshields W, Fielding S 1985 What every woman should know. New Generation 4(1)

Harris R E 1970 An evaluation of the median episiotomy American Journal of Obstetrics and Gynecology 106: 660–665

House M J et al 1987 Episiotomy and the perineum: a random controlled trial. Journal of Obstetrics and Gynaecology 7(2): 107–110

Lane P 1990 The controversial art (episiotomy). Parents (May): 77–78

Nolan M 1989 Episiotomy and perineal repair (a summary 1984–1989). New Generation (Sept): 24–26

Paciornik M 1990 Commentary: arguments against episiotomy and in favour of squatting for birth. Birth 17(2): 104–105

Sherriff J 1984 Think before you cut. Nursing Mirror 158(11): ix–xii

Sleep J, Grant A 1987 West Berkshire perineal management trial: three-year follow-up. British Medical Journal 295: 749–751

Sleep J, Grant A 1987 Pelvic floor exercises in post-natal care. Midwifery 3: 158–164

Snooks S J et al 1985 Risk factors in childbirth causing damage to the pelvic floor innervation. British Journal of Surgery (suppl) 72: 515–517

Reference centres

Birthright, 27 Sussex Place, Regent's Park, London NW1 4SP

National Childbirth Trust, 9 Queensborough Terrace, Bayswater, London W2 3TB (071-221-3822)

4 The bladder and urethra

(Plate 2A and B, Plate 3B)

The situation, shape and size of the bladder will vary according to the amount of urine it contains.

Situation The empty bladder lies in the pelvic cavity with its base resting on the upper half of the vagina and its apex directed towards the symphysis pubis. As it fills with urine it rises up and out of the pelvic cavity to become an abdominal organ and can be palpated above the symphysis pubis when full. As it rises it displaces the body of the uterus.

Shape When empty it is pyramidal but as it fills with urine it becomes globular.

Size The bladder can accommodate about 300 ml of urine before the desire to micturate is experienced. It is capable of retaining a very much greater volume.

Gross structure (Fig. 4.1)

The trigone is the base of the bladder. It is directed backwards and downwards and is separated from the upper half of the vaginal wall by connective tissue. Unlike the main body of the bladder, the trigone is not capable of distension and it remains 'flat'.

The apex points upwards and forwards towards the symphysis pubis. From it the urachus continues upwards to the umbilicus. The **urachus** is the fibrosed remnant of the embryonic yolk sac.

The neck is continuous with the urethra, and is the area at the junction of bladder and urethra.

The superior surface (fundus) is triangular in shape and is almost entirely covered with peritoneum. Posteriorly, where it is reflected up and over the body of the uterus, it is loosely attached and lies in folds. This arrangement of peritoneum allows the essential movement of both bladder and uterus. The pouch of peritoneum is described as the **uterovesical pouch**.

Microscopic structure
(excluding the trigone)

Transitional epithelium, which has characteristic features of distension, contraction and impermeability to water, is the mucous membrane lining of the

67

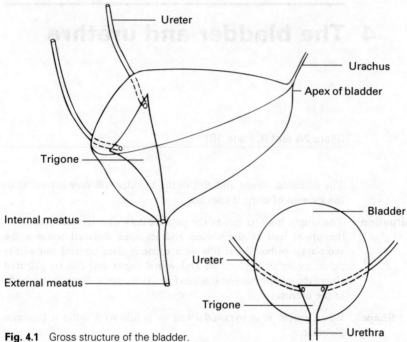

Fig. 4.1 Gross structure of the bladder.

bladder. It is arranged in folds, the **rugae**, to allow for bladder distension.

Connective tissue is areolar in type.

Muscle is non-striated (sometimes synonymously named plain or smooth or involuntary muscle). It is the type of muscle found in many body organs where slow, continued, automatic responses are required. It is arranged in three layers: a middle layer of circular fibres lies between inner and outer layers of longitudinal fibres. Nevertheless, there is much intermingling of the fibres in each layer and the layers can by no means be strictly differentiated. The muscle in the body of the bladder is called the **detrusor muscle**.

Peritoneum covers the superior surface of the bladder. Its arrangement has already been described.

The trigone (Fig. 4.2) This is also called the base of the bladder and is triangular in shape, each side of the triangle measuring 2.5 cm in length when the bladder is contracted. In the distended bladder the measurement may be increased to 5 cm. Entering obliquely at the lateral angles are the **ureters** which pass through the bladder wall for a distance of 2 cm. They raise the epithelial lining as they pass through. This helps to prevent urine from regurgitating back into the ureter when the bladder is full because there is compression of the raised tissues. The **urethra** leaves the third orifice at the neck of the bladder.

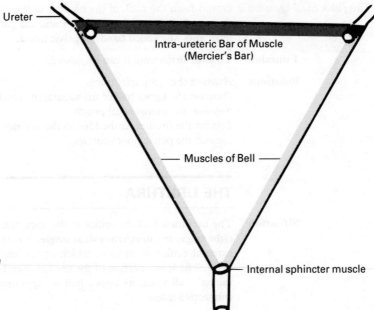

Ureter

Intra-ureteric Bar of Muscle
(Mercier's Bar)

Muscles of Bell

Fig. 4.2 Trigone of the
bladder.

Internal sphincter muscle

Transitional epithelium lines the trigone, but it lies smoothly with no rugae, for this area, unlike the bladder, does not expand.

Connective tissue is areolar in type.

Muscle **Mercier's bar**, or the intraureteric bar, is the muscle lying between the ureteric orifices. When the bar of muscle contracts during micturition it compresses still further the raised tissues in the site of the ureteric orifices and closes them so that urine does not flow back into the ureters. This is non-striated muscle.

Bell's muscles, also non-striated, extend between each ureteric orifice and the internal meatus of the urethra. They continue into the muscle wall of the urethra for half its length. They play a part in the opening of the internal meatus when the urethrovesical angle changes at the onset of micturition and they direct the flow of urine into the urethral lumen.

Blood supply Blood supply is via inferior and superior vesical arteries from the internal iliac artery. Venous drainage is by corresponding veins.

Lymphatic drainage Lymphatic drainage is into the external iliac glands.

Nerve supply Nerve supply is from the sympathetic and parasympathetic nerves from the Lee–Frankenhäuser plexus (now more commonly known as the sacral plexus).

Supports The neck of the bladder rests on the **pubococcygeus muscle**. The **urachus** extends from the apex of the bladder to the umbilicus.

Two lateral ligaments extend from the side walls of the pelvis to the side walls of the bladder.

Two pubovesical ligaments extend from the neck of the bladder to the pubic bodies. They are the true ligaments of the bladder and are part of the pubocervical ligaments, thickened bands of pelvic fascia.

Function To store urine until it can be voided.

Relations *Anterior:* the symphysis pubis
Posterior: the upper half of the vagina; the cervix
Superior: the uterovesical pouch
Inferior: the urethra, embedded in the anterior vaginal wall
Lateral: the pelvic floor muscles.

THE URETHRA

Situation The urethra leaves the orifice at the apex of the trigone almost at a right angle, the **urethrovesical angle**. It extends from there to the external orifice or meatus, which opens into the vestibule of the vulva. The lower portion of the urethra is embedded in the anterior vaginal wall while its upper half is separated from the vagina by connective tissue.

Shape The female urethra is slightly S-shaped and is tubular with blind crypts opening out from it. These are remnants of the embryonic prostate gland. The lowest ones, known as **Skene's ducts**, are not blind but turn downwards and open on each side of the urethral orifice in the vestibule.

Size The female urethra is much shorter than that of the male. It is 4 cm in length but is capable of considerable elongation. The diameter of its lumen is 6 mm but this can easily be dilated with a urinary catheter.

Gross structure (Fig. 4.3)

The internal meatus lies at the junction of the urethra and bladder.

The external meatus is the urethral orifice which opens into the vestibule. It lies about 2.5 cm below the clitoris.

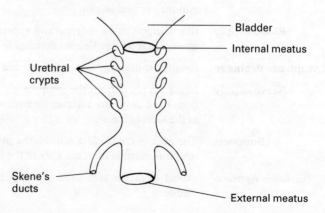

Bladder
Internal meatus
Urethral crypts
Skene's ducts
External meatus

Fig. 4.3 Gross structure of the urethra.

The urethral crypts are the blind ducts opening from the urethral wall.

Skene's ducts are the two lowest ducts which open into the vestibule.

Microscopic structure

Stratified epithelium, a modified skin, forms a protective lining for the distal half of the urethra.

Transitional epithelium, like that in the bladder, lines the proximal half.

Connective tissue

Muscle There is an **inner layer of longitudinal fibres**. Some of these fibres are a continuation of the muscles of Bell and extend halfway down the urethra. The rest are a continuation of the detrusor muscle.

There is an **outer layer of circular fibres**, some of which are arranged as spirals. This layer is also partly composed of fibres from the detrusor muscle.

Sphincters The **internal sphincter** has an internal and external portion and makes a loop around the neck of the bladder at the internal meatus. Some muscle fibres extend into the pubococcygeus muscle, one of the deep muscles of the pelvic floor. The meatus is opened for micturition by the muscles of Bell.

The **external sphincter** lies between the superficial and deep muscle layers of the pelvic floor, at the distal end of the urethra. It is also known as the **compressor urethrae** or **sphincter of the membranous urethra**. This sphincter also has two parts:

1. *Involuntary circular muscle fibres* which form a true sphincter
2. *Transverse voluntary fibres* which contract to expel the last few millilitres of urine from the bladder.

The **middle third** of the urethra has many intermingling fibres of elastic tissue, collagen and fascia with involuntary circular fibres of the urethral muscle and voluntary fibres of the pubococcygeus muscle. This results in there being greater intraurethral pressure in its middle third and this is of importance in maintaining continence of urine. The area acts as a sphincter and contracts to prevent involuntary passing of urine when a woman coughs, sneezes or laughs.

Blood supply Blood supply is from the inferior vesical artery and the pudendal artery. Venous drainage is by corresponding veins.

Lymphatic drainage Lymphatic drainage is into the internal iliac glands.

Nerve supply Nerve supply is from sympathetic nerves to the internal sphincter muscles. The external sphincter is under voluntary control and is supplied by the pudendal nerve.

Supports
1. *The anterior vaginal wall*: The whole urethra is supported by fibromuscular tissue from the pubococcygeus muscle
2. *Other structures of the pelvic floor.*

Function   The urethra is the canal through which urine is eliminated from the body.

MAINTENANCE OF CONTINENCE

Bladder muscle tone

1. Although urine is passing continuously down the ureters into the bladder, the amount being retained normally distends the bladder very slowly. This makes it possible for the detrusor muscle to remain in a state of 'controlled' relaxation.

2. Intravesical pressure is accordingly not increased until, on average, about 300 ml of urine cause so much distension that receptors in the bladder wall are stimulated.

3. Then there is an urge to micturate as the detrusor muscles start to contract.

Intraurethral pressure

This is brought about by the urethrovesical angle, as previously described, and closes the upper part of the urethra. The urethral walls lie in apposition. The middle third of the urethra has many intermingling fibres of elastic tissue, collagen, fascia, involuntary muscle fibres of urethral muscle and voluntary fibres of the pubococcygeus muscle. This provides much greater intraurethral pressure than in the upper and lower thirds. The walls are almost 'squeezed ' together and this is of major importance in maintaining continence of urine. The middle third of the urethra acts like a sphincter and contracts to prevent the involuntary passing of urine when intra-abdominal pressure is increased by such acts as laughing, sneezing or coughing.

Sphincter control

This is now believed to play a much less significant part than was thought in previous years, but involuntary fibres of the internal and external meatus remain contracted while voluntary muscles of the external sphincter are in a similar state.

PHYSIOLOGY OF MICTURITION

When the bladder can no longer accommodate urine without intravesical pressure being increased (usually at a volume of about 300 ml), receptors in the bladder wall initiate contractions of the detrusor muscle. In infants, micturition occurs involuntarily and immediately. In adults, the deed can be delayed until the time and place are appropriate. Should the sensory stimulus be delayed for too long, however, it will be referred as pain.

With initiation of the contractions of detrusor muscle, relaxation of the pubococcygeus muscle takes place and there is a reduction of urethral support resulting in the following sequence of events:

1. The internal meatus opens
2. The uterovesical angle alters
3. The upper part of the urethra fills with urine
4. Urine acts as an irritant on the urethral walls
5. The detrusor muscle contracts more strongly
6. Urine is forced down the urethra as intra-abdominal pressure is increased
7. The external sphincter opens
8. Urine is voided until the bladder is empty.

Interruption of the flow of urine is possible because the pubococcygeus muscle is under voluntary control:

• The pubococcygeus muscle is contracted during the flow
• The bladder is drawn up
• The urethra is elongated
• The external sphincter muscle is fixed in contraction.

When the pubococcygeus is relaxed again, the cycle of events just described is automatically re-commenced.

URINARY DISORDERS

The bladder is closely related to the rectum as well as to the organs of the genital tract and all organs are supplied by nerves from the sacral plexus. In pregnancy also, because of the developing fetus, they are all competing for decreasing space in the pelvis. As one organ enlarges another is compressed, and it is therefore not unusual for disturbances of micturition to occur in pregnancy and labour as well as during the postnatal period.

In pregnancy

Increased frequency   In the first 12 weeks of pregnancy, while the enlarging uterus is still a pelvic organ, the bladder requires to be emptied at more frequent intervals because there is less room for it to expand. This type of increased frequency is said to be **physiological**. During the last 4 weeks of pregnancy, when the fetal head lies in the pelvis, there is a recurrence of increased frequency for the same reason. In the middle weeks of pregnancy, increased frequency arising in association with **dysuria** is due to **urinary infection**. This commonly arises between the 16th and 24th weeks of pregnancy, and is a difficult condition to cure at this time. It may recur throughout pregnancy and the puerperium. About 2% of pregnant women are affected.

Acute retention   This is a rare complication of pregnancy but sometimes occurs at about the 12th week of gestation if the uterus is retroverted. The uterus cannot rise out of the pelvis beyond the hollow of the sacrum if the bladder is full and the uterus therefore becomes impacted. This is a vicious circle: the uterus cannot rise out of the pelvis until the bladder is emptied, but the bladder cannot be spontaneously emptied because it is nipped between the symphysis pubis and the enlarged uterus. The treatment lies in passing a urinary catheter and slowly draining the bladder, after which there are rarely any further complications because the uterus can then stand erect and rise out of the pelvic cavity.

Stress incontinence   Urine is sometimes passed involuntarily towards the end of pregnancy if the fetal head is deeply engaged in the pelvis. Small amounts of urine may be passed if the patient coughs, sneezes or laughs. Incontinence of urine should not be confused with early rupture of membranes. In order to make a differential diagnosis, the pH should be determined. Urine has a pH of 5.3–6.0, while amniotic fluid is alkaline.

In labour

Increased frequency   This occurs most commonly in association with the occipitoposterior position of the fetal head. The occiput of the deflexed head applies increased pressure on the nerves of the sacral plexus and with the consequential increased stimulus of sensory receptors in the bladder wall, the woman has a more frequent desire to micturate. It is sometimes an almost continual desire even though intravesical pressure is not increased. Only very small amounts of urine are passed at each attempt.

Acute retention   1. *Pressure on the sacral plexus from the fetal head* may conversely cause poor stimulus and the motor impulses which stimulate muscle activity are depressed. Intravesical pressure rises but even though the bladder is overdistended the woman feels no desire to micturate. If the bladder becomes overdistended, nerve receptors in the bladder wall can also be inhibited and the woman has no desire to micturate even though intravesical pressure is raised.

2. *Pressure on the neck of the bladder and urethra from the fetal head* causes compression of those structures and exerts extra-urethral pressure. Mechanically it is now impossible to pass urine since the internal meatus and urethrovesical angle are compressed. The bladder becomes distended with urine and its retention is now exacerbated because there is lack of nervous stimulus from receptors. The neck of the bladder is nipped between the fetal head and the symphysis pubis.

3. *Anaesthesia*   Epidural or caudal block temporarily paralyse the nerves which supply the bladder. Sympathetic efferent nerve fibres from the lowest two thoracic and the first two lumbar segments of the spinal cord and parasympathetic efferent fibres from the 2nd, 3rd and 4th sacral segments are all 'blocked'. The woman receiving this type of analgesia will not be aware that her bladder is full.

Effects of a full bladder in labour

- *Delays descent of the fetal head,* the commonest cause of such a delay in multigravid women
- *Reduces efficiency of uterine contractions* in all three stages
- *There is a dribbling of urine* with each expulsive contraction during the second stage
- *Compression* of the bladder by the fetal head causes *bruising and oedema of bladder and urethra*
- *Causes unnecessary pain*
- *Delays delivery of the placenta*
- *Predisposes to postpartum haemorrhage* by inhibiting uterine contractions
- *Can cause vesicovaginal fistula* if trauma is severe or pressure is prolonged
- Over-distension of the bladder *can cause later detrusor instability.*

It is therefore essential that the woman should empty her bladder early in the first stage of labour and then every 2 hours subsequently. If, when routine observations are being made, the filling bladder can be palpated above the symphysis pubis, then the woman should be reminded to go to the lavatory. Should she be unable to pass urine, then the bladder must be emptied by catheterisation but this should be avoided if at all possible because:

- There is always a risk of subsequent urinary infection
- There is a possible risk of trauma to the elongated urethra with its narrowed lumen.

In the puerperium

Increased frequency

Physiological factors   During the first 48 hours of the puerperium there is an increased diuresis as the result of: (1) a reduction in the mother's blood volume; (2) autolysis of uterine muscle fibre. The mother therefore finds it necessary to pass urine more frequently.

Infection   There may be a recurrence of antenatal urinary tract infection or it may arise during the puerperium for the first time. The lochia, tissue trauma and stasis of urine are all contributory factors, offering a medium in which pathogenic bacteria flourish. Preventive measures include regular and complete emptying of the bladder and strict perianal hygiene. Any perineal suture line should be kept as dry as possible; the use of tissues following urination will be found helpful in this matter. The causative infecting organism is most commonly *Escherichia coli.*

Muscle tone   Laxity of pelvic floor muscle tone, or prolonged compression of nerve fibres during labour, results in contraction of the detrusor muscle before the normal intravesical pressure is reached. This low filling level of the bladder, occurring in addition to the physiological increased diuresis, exacerbates the desire to micturate more frequently.

Acute retention of urine   This may be the result of:

1. *Posture*: If the mother is confined to bed and must use a bedpan, the unaccustomed position for micturition often causes difficulty. In most instances, transfer to a Sani-chair will solve the problem.

2. *Embarrassment*: Where there is lack of privacy, especially when the mother knows that she can be heard micturating, motor impulses may be inhibited.

3. *Fear of pain*: Especially in the presence of perineal or vaginal grazes, a bruised perineum or perineal sutures.

4. *Atony of bladder muscle*: Over-distension of the bladder during labour or prolonged pressure of the fetal head can cause diminution of bladder stimulus since both nerves and motor impulses can be impaired.

5. *Elongation of the urethra*: Together with bruising and/or oedema occlude the lumen of the urethra.

Acute retention of urine always causes some degree of bladder muscle and detrusor instability. This increases the likelihood of stress incontinence occurring in subsequent pregnancies.

Retention with overflow
(overflow incontinence)

1. *Consequence of acute retention*   The bladder is not capable of unlimited distension and if the desire to empty it is inhibited, urine will dribble away intermittently because the internal meatus cannot remain closed when the bladder muscle tone becomes greater than the intraurethral tone.

2. *Muscle tone*   As a result of atony due to a long or difficult labour, the lax pelvic floor and bladder muscles allow the base of the bladder to become convex and lean towards the anterior vaginal wall. Urine 'pools' in the convexity, making it impossible for urine to be completely voided – that in the 'pool' is retained.

3. *Full bladder in labour*   If the bladder is not emptied at the end of the first stage, there is a dribbling of urine with each expulsive contraction during the second stage. An attempt should be made to empty the bladder by passing a urinary catheter.

Incontinence   True incontinence of urine associated with midwifery practice is rarely seen in this country today unless a patient is unconscious or has suffered a spinal injury. In underdeveloped countries it is more common because deliveries are often unattended and skilled obstetric facilities are unavailable in many areas. The condition results from a major degree of trauma such as a vesico- or urethrovaginal fistula.

Much more commonly in this country the complication of stress incontinence is seen.

Stress incontinence   As described earlier, urinary continence is maintained in three ways.

1. *Muscle tone of the bladder* (detrusor muscle), which controls intravesical pressure.

2. *Intraurethral pressure* provided by the pubococcygeus muscle and intermingling mixed fibres of the middle third of the urethra.

3. *Sphincter control*, including here, although it is not a true sphincter, the urethrovesical angle at the neck of the bladder. This angle, which closes the internal meatus, is under the control of the pelvic floor muscles.

These three factors combine to prevent the involuntary passing of urine when intra-abdominal pressure is increased by laughing, sneezing or coughing. The major factor now believed to maintain urinary continence is the good tone of the muscles of the anterior pelvic floor rather than the sphincter muscles.

These muscles and the nerves which serve them (pudendal nerve and branches of the sacral plexus) are particularly susceptible to stress and trauma during childbirth when they are stretched and compressed. Trauma to the nerves reduces the power of the already overstretched and weakened muscles that they supply, although in most healthy women who exercise regularly muscle tone is soon regained. The primigravid patient who commences labour with all her muscles in good tone is the least likely to be troubled with stress incontinence. But with subsequent deliveries the structures are subject to repeated stress and the incidence of stress incontinence increases with parity. The incidence is also higher in older women (partly due to hormonal changes) and those who have been subject to prolonged labours and/or instrumental delivery.

Urge incontinence   This is an involuntary loss of urine accompanied simultaneously by a strong urge to micturate. It is caused by unstable detrusor muscle, lax pelvic floor muscles, cystocele or urinary infection.

Prophylaxis

Antenatal   Maintenance of good pelvic floor muscle tone by:

- Teaching perineal awareness
- Encouraging the woman to participate in exercise such as walking and swimming, if she is not already doing so
- Assessment of pelvic floor muscle tone in multigravidae as previously described and consideration of elective caesarean section for those women at risk.

In labour
- An awareness by the midwife of the need to avoid overstretching of pelvic floor muscles during delivery
- Awareness by the midwife of the need to remind the woman to empty her bladder regularly during the first stage and to ensure that the bladder is empty at the onset of the second stage
- The use of episiotomy or forceps delivery when necessary to shorten the duration of the second stage (episiotomy, pudendal nerve block and spinal anaesthetic are not associated of themselves with nerve injury)
- The use of caesarean section in selected women where there is the risk of increased damage to an already incompetent pelvic floor.

Puerperium

Exercise As in the antenatal period, pelvic floor exercises are valuable in strengthening these muscles but of greater importance is the participation in activities which improve the tone of all muscle – swimming, dancing, keep fit, aerobics etc.

Postnatal specific care of the bladder

The mother should be encouraged to empty her bladder before she leaves the labour ward. If she cannot do so, reminders should be given hourly during the first few (daytime) hours until she passes urine.

In many obstetric units urinary output is recorded for at least the first 24 hours after delivery to exclude bladder atony.

The mother can be quite unaware that her bladder is full and daily abdominal palpation will exclude the retention of urine if she is passing only small amounts. A full bladder will displace the uterus and also cause subinvolution. It is therefore important to exclude retention of urine with overflow.

At the postnatal clinic 6 weeks following delivery, the special investigations relating to the function of the bladder and micturition include the diagnosis of increased frequency of urine, stress urgency to micturate, stress incontinence of urine, urethrocele and cystocele. The patient must be referred for follow-up care where appropriate.

A survey carried out in 1983 by the National Childbirth Trust is referred to in Chapter 3. It should be read again here in association with the subject matter of this chapter.

The report of a small but interesting trial of treatment for women suffering stress urinary incontinence was published in October 1988. Weighted vaginal cones were used to exercise the pelvic muscles as an alternative to treatment by electrical stimulation, physiotherapy, pessaries or surgery. 70% of women felt their condition to be improved or cured and 90% found it an acceptable form of treatment. The report is listed in the bibliography for this chapter.

Table 4.1 A summary of urinary complications

In pregnancy	Increased frequency	Physiological Infection
	Acute retention	Increased retroverted uterus
	Stress incontinence	Laxity of pelvic floor muscles Pregnancy hormones Position of fetal head
In labour	Increased frequency	Occipitoposterior position
	Acute retention	Spinal anaesthesia Pressure on sacral plexus Pressure on bladder
	Retention with overflow	
In puerperium	Increased frequency	Physiological Infection Lax muscle tone
	Acute retention	Posture Embarrassment Pain Elongation of urethra Spinal anaesthesia
	Retention with overflow	Acute retention Lax muscle tone
	Incontinence	Trauma
	Stress incontinence	Lax pelvic floor muscles Nerve damage Poor bladder tone Poor sphincter control

REVISION QUESTIONS

Describe the anatomy of the female bladder and urethra. Why is it important that a midwife should have this knowledge?

Describe the urethra. Discuss the obstetric indications for catheterisation of the bladder.

Describe the urethra and its relations. Under what conditions may retention of urine occur during pregnancy, labour and the puerperium?

Describe the female bladder and urethra. How may these structures be affected by pregnancy and labour?

Describe the urinary bladder. What disturbances of micturition may occur during pregnancy, labour and the puerperium?

Describe the anatomy of the bladder. How may urinary infections be avoided in pregnancy, labour and the puerperium?

Describe the physiology of micturition. What disturbances of micturition may occur within the postnatal period?

A woman delivered 12 hours previously is unable to pass urine. List the possible causes and describe the management and care given by the midwife.

Describe the physiology of micturition. What disturbances of micturition may occur during the puerperium? How may they be recognised and treated?

Outline the physiology of micturition. What disorders of micturition may occur and how may they be managed during the antenatal period, labour and the first week of puerperium?

Write short notes on:

- Problems of micturition in the puerperium
- Causes, prevention and treatment of stress incontinence
- Causes of acute retention of urine in the puerperium
- Causes and treatment of urinary disorders in pregnancy
- The importance of pelvic floor structures in the maintenance of urinary continence.

REFERENCES AND FURTHER READING

Books and reports

Junor P (ed) 1988 What every woman needs to know: facts and fears about pregnancy, childbirth and womanhood. Century, London

Polden M, Mantle J 1990 Physiotherapy in obstetrics and gynaecology. Butterworth-Heinemann, London

Webb C 1986 Women's health: midwifery and gynaecological nursing. Hodder Education. (ed Norton C), ch 6

Articles

Blannin J P 1989 The sooner the better! Teaching continence promotion to women. Professional Nurse (Dec): 149–150

Cardozo L 1990 Female urinary incontinence. Update (March 1): 481–490

Dolman M 1989 Are you asking the right questions? New Generation (June): 20–21

Gordon H, Cogue M 1985 Perineal muscle function after childbirth. Lancet ii: 123–125

Greenshields W, Fielding S 1985 What every woman should know (prolapse). New Generation 4(4): 9

Greenshields W, Fielding S 1983 Prolapse survey. New Generation 2(2): 3

Henalla S M et al 1989 Non-operative methods in the treatment of genuine stress incontinence. Journal of Obstetrics and Gynaecology 9(3): 222–225

Henry N M et al 1982 The pelvic floor in the descending perineum syndrome. British Journal of Surgery 69: 470–472

Hilton P 1988 Urinary incontinence during sexual intercourse: a common but rarely volunteered symptom. British Journal of Obstetrics and Gynaecology 95(4): 377–381

Kegal A H 1986 Early genital relaxation. New techniques of diagnosis and non-surgical treatment. Journal of Obstetrics and Gynaecology 8: 515–520

Landon C R 1990 Mechanical properties of fascia during pregnancy: a possible factor in the development of stress incontinence of urine. Contemporary Reviews in Obstetrics and Gynaecology (Jan): 40–46

Langley T 1989 Educating Anne (health education approach to stress incontinence). Nursing Times (June): 9–10

Middleburgh L, Staples S 1988 Physiotherapy symposium on incontinence and its management, London, October 1987. ACPOG Journal 63: 15–18

Montgomery E 1986 Promoting continence: pelvic power community outlook. Nursing Times 82.37: 33–34

Peattie A B et al 1988 Vaginal cones: a conservative method of treating genuine stress incontinence. British Journal of Obstetrics and Gynaecology 95: 1049–1053

Schuessler B, Hesse U, Dimpfl T, Anthuber C 1988 Epidural anaesthesia and avoidance of post partum stress urinary incontinence. Lancet i: 762

Shepherd A M 1983 Management of urinary incontinence: prevention or cure. Physiotherapy 69: 109–110

Smith A R B et al 1989 The role of pudendal nerve damage in the aetiology of genuine stress incontinence in women. British Journal of Obstetrics and Gynaecology 96(1): 29–32

Snooks S J et al 1985 Risk factors in childbirth causing damage to the pelvic floor innervation. British Journal of Surgery (suppl) 72: 515–517

Swash M 1988 Childbirth and incontinence. Midwifery 4(1): 13–18

Tapp A, Cardozo L, Versi E, Montgomery J, Studd J 1988 The effect of vaginal delivery on the urethral sphincter. British Journal of Obstetrics and Gynaecology 95(2): 142–146

5 The external genital organs

(Plate 5A and B)

The external genital organs of the female (Fig. 5.1) are known collectively as the vulva and include the following structures:

Mons veneris A pad of fatty tissue, covered by skin, which lies over the symphysis pubis. After puberty, a growth of hair develops on it.

Labia majora (sing. labium majus) Two large rounded folds of fatty tissue covered by skin which meet anteriorly at the mons veneris. As they pass backwards towards the anus they become flatter and merge into the perineal body. The terminal portions of the round ligaments are inserted into the fatty tissue. The inner aspects of the labia are smooth and contain numerous sweat and sebaceous glands while their outer aspects, after puberty, are covered with hair.

Labia minora (sing. labium minus) Two smaller folds of pink skin lying longitudinally within the labia majora. They are smooth, having no covering of hair, but do contain a few sweat and sebaceous glands. The area they enclose is known as the **vestibule**. Each labium minus divides into two folds anteriorly. The upper folds surround the **clitoris** and unite to form the **prepuce**. The two lower folds are attached to the undersurface of the clitoris and are known as the **frenulum**. Posteriorly, the labia

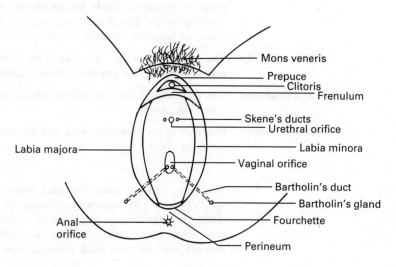

Mons veneris
Prepuce
Clitoris
Frenulum
Skene's ducts
Urethral orifice
Labia majora
Labia minora
Vaginal orifice
Bartholin's duct
Bartholin's gland
Anal orifice
Fourchette
Perineum

Fig. 5.1 External genital organs.

minora unite to form a thin fold of skin, the **fourchette**, which is torn when a first-degree perineal tear is sustained during delivery.

The clitoris   A small, extremely sensitive, erectile structure, situated, as previously explained, within the folds of the prepuce and frenulum. It is composed of two bodies, the corpora cavernosa, which lie side by side and extend backwards to be attached to the periosteum of the bodies of the pubic bones. The clitoris is a structure which may be compared with the male penis but, unlike the penis, does not transmit the urethra.

We are now living in a multiracial society where there is a wide range of different religions, beliefs and cultural practices. Female circumcision is a traditional practice of which we, in the UK, are now becoming much more aware. It affects the appearance and function of the vulva in relation to the degree in which it is practised. Further details will be found at the end of this chapter.

The vestibule   In order to observe the vestibule, the folds of the labia must be separated to bring it into view. There are six openings into it:

The urethral meatus   Known also as the external orifice of the urethra, this lies 2.5 cm below the clitoris.

Two Skene's ducts   The openings of Skene's tubules which run parallel with the urethra for about 6 mm, and then open, one on each side of the urethral orifice.

The vaginal orifice   Also known as the **introitus**, this occupies the lower two-thirds of the vestibule. In a virgin it is covered by the hymen, a thin perforated membrane through which the menstrual flow can pass. The hymen is ruptured following intercourse and further laceration occurs during childbirth, the remaining tags of skin being known as **carunculae myrtiformes**.

Two Bartholin's ducts and glands   The glands lie on each side of the vagina, resting on the triangular ligaments. About the size and shape of haricot beans, they are composed of racemose glands and secrete mucus. The ducts are the openings of the glands and open outside the hymen so that the glandular secretion keeps the external genitalia moist.

Blood supply   The pudendal arteries, branches of the femoral artery, supply the external genitals. Venous drainage is by the corresponding veins.

Lymphatic drainage   Some drainage is into the inguinal glands and some is into the external iliac glands.

Nerve supply   Branches of the pudendal nerve and the perineal nerve provide the nerve supply.

The vulva becomes very distended towards the end of the first stage of labour and even more so during the second stage when the fetal head is descending quite rapidly. A practical knowledge of the basic anatomy of these parts is therefore essential in order that the midwife can carry out such procedures as catheterisation of the bladder and episiotomy with the maximum of efficiency and minimum of trauma to her patient.

COLLECTION OF URINE SPECIMENS

Because of the proximity of the urethral, vaginal and rectal orifices, *Escherichia coli*, normal inhabitants of the rectum, have easy access to the urethra. The organisms flourish on blood from menstrual loss or on the lochia. All female children should therefore be taught the importance of correct rectal and perineal cleansing, i.e. cleansing in an anteroposterior direction. Such instruction should be reinforced during the ante- and postnatal periods. **Cystitis is said to occur in about 2% of women, sometimes being asymptomatic**.

When the laboratory is asked to test a specimen of urine for culture and deposits, it is now more usual to collect a clean (i.e. midstream) specimen rather than a catheter specimen because of the risk of infecting the urinary tract when a catheter is introduced into the bladder.

Midstream specimen After considerable research into various techniques, it has been has demonstrated that when a woman *bends forward* and stands astride the lavatory, her urine passes directly downwards, without passing the vaginal or rectal orifices. A midstream specimen collected in this way into a sterile container is therefore uncontaminated.

Suffice it to say that every department will have its own standard procedure. Whatever the method, the woman should be very clearly instructed in the technique so that her urine is not contaminated by her hands, any vaginal discharge or the perineal and perianal areas.

About 60 ml in midstream should be collected into a sterile jug, or a sterile specimen bottle should be filled directly if the specimen is to go to the laboratory. It should be accompanied by the completed and signed request form and despatched immediately unless it can be stored in a cool place (4°C) where any organisms that the specimen contains will not proliferate.

Catheterisation of the bladder There are a few occasions when of necessity a catheter must be passed into the bladder because the patient cannot pass urine voluntarily. The following are occasions when a catheter is used.

Antenatal period An incarcerated, retroverted, pregnant uterus cannot rise out of the pelvis and therefore interferes with bladder function (see Ch. 4).

In labour During the first or second stages of labour, the descending fetal head may interfere with bladder function. If the bladder is not emptied, trauma may occur. A full bladder in the third stage of labour should always be emptied, as it affects uterine action and can cause retained placenta and postpartum haemorrhage.

If catheterisation is being performed during labour, it will be found necessary to insert a greater length of catheter than when the procedure is being carried out in the ante- or postnatal periods.

This is because the bladder is drawn up into the abdomen during labour and the urethra is elongated and narrowed.

In the puerperium

1. **Acute retention of urine** is less common now that early ambulation of patients is practised, but it does occur from time to time.

2. **Retention with overflow** is another occasional complication, and is a condition in which the bladder is not emptied when the patient urinates, the amount of residual urine is .therefore increased daily.

3. **True incontinence** occurs, rarely, as a result of prolonged and difficult labour, and as a consequence of trauma the urine is bloodstained. In this condition a self-retaining catheter should be inserted and left in situ at least until the urine is clear.

Catheterisation should never be carried out unless it is absolutely necessary and when this necessity does arise it should be a sterile procedure undertaken with scrupulous care.

INSPECTION OF THE VULVA

The vulva should always be carefully inspected when abdominal palpation or vaginal examination is being made, whether this be antenatally, in labour or following the birth of the infant.
Abnormalities that might be revealed include:

1. *Pruritus vulvae.* Intense irritation felt by the woman may be the result of **glycosuria** or **moniliasis**. Diagnostic tests are made on urine and a vaginal swab. The vulva is red and scratching may have caused a skin infection.

2. *Varicose veins.* More often seen in multigravidae, or women with hydramnios or multiple pregnancy. They are caused partly by the venous return being impeded and exacerbated by the relaxation of blood vessel walls brought about by progesterone and by the increased volume of circulating blood. They can be very painful and treatment lies partly in the application of a firm perineal pad to give support while advising the woman to rest in the recumbent position as much as possible. There is a danger that they may rupture. The condition is associated with varicosities of the lower limbs, haemorrhoids and oedema.

3. *Oedema.* Associated with varicose veins of the vulva, oedema is seen more commonly in association with pre-eclampsia. The treatment is of that condition. Where unilateral oedema of one labium is present, the inner surface should be examined to exclude a **syphilitic chancre**.

4. *Vulval warts.* Are most commonly associated with a viral infection and they can spread profusely during pregnancy. They are sometimes associated with a **trichomoniasis** infection. Vulval warts are also associated with **gonorrhoea** or they nay be **syphilitic condylomata**. Differential diagnosis must be made and the

appropriate treatment then prescribed (see Ch. 6: sexually transmitted diseases)

5. *Vulval swellings* are most often associated with a blocked Bartholin's duct or infected **Bartholin's gland**. Gonorrhoea as a cause of a **Bartholin's abscess** must be excluded but is not the only cause.

6. *Vulval sore or herpes genitalis* is caused by **herpes simplex virus** or the **syphilitic chancre**. Both require diagnosis and specific treatment.

7. *Vulval haematoma* arises shortly after completion of labour. Bleeding into the subcutaneous tissues of the vulva and/or vaginal wall is caused by ruptured blood vessels. It may be due to the trauma of pressure or be associated with the repair of a perineal tear or episiotomy. The newly delivered mother complains of pain and is likely to suffer a degree of shock not related to the size of the haematoma. Blood transfusion is necessary to counteract more severe shock and haemorrhage. Unless very small and causing minor symptoms, the haematoma will need to be drained and the area re-sutured, usually under general anaesthetic. This lady will be very frightened and as well as medical treatment needs companionship and reassurance while she is awaiting surgery.

8. *Vulval scars*. The most common scarring which is seen during vulval examination is the scarring of the perineum due to a healed episiotomy scar but anterior scarring is associated with rupture of the tissues where female circumcision has been performed.

FEMALE CIRCUMCISION

The practice of female circumcision, which always involves, at the least, incision of the prepuce, is not limited to puberty rites among primitive and uneducated people. It is considered an essential requisite for marriage by many ethnic groups in over 20 African countries, by the Moslems of Oman, South Yemen and the United Arab Emirates and by Moslem groups in Indonesia and Malaysia. Intensive campaigns have been conducted in Africa to stamp out the practice but legislation is useless where it cannot be enforced. Middle-class Arabic parents in particular appear anxious to preserve this tradition of 'ritual cleansing' not just for social, cultural and religious reasons but to preserve their family honour. Recent news reports (1988) indicate that Harley Street consultants have been approached by Arab women with requests for this operation to be performed. Carried out as a hospital procedure under medical supervision, at least the effects of physical shock and the complications of subsequent haemorrhage and genitourinary infection are minimised.

Three different types of female circumcision are practised:

1. *Circumcision* (termed **sunna** by Moslems): The fold of the labia minora termed the prepuce is cut. This is the least traumatic

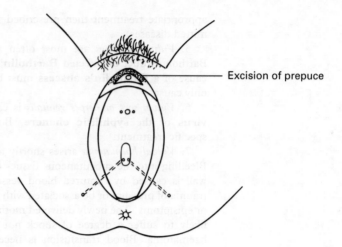

Excision of prepuce

Fig. 5.2 Clitoridectomy.

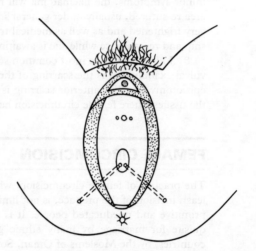

Fig. 5.3 Excision – shading indicates the excised structures.

of the three types and is the only method which can be truly termed circumcision. Unfortunately, it is the method least practised.

2. *Excision* (Fig. 5.3): Part, or the whole, of the labia minora is excised, together with the clitoris.

3. *Infibulation* (Fig. 5.4): The clitoris, the labia minora and at least the anterior two-thirds of the labia majora are excised. The lateral walls of the vulva are then stitched together (using thorns in a primitive society) leaving only a small orifice for the passage of urine and the menstrual flow. The orifice is widened prior to the consummation of marriage.

Both excision and infibulation will give rise to soft-tissue damage during vaginal delivery.

With the emigration or 'extended' visits of African and/or Moslem women to the UK, a midwife will quite possibly, during her

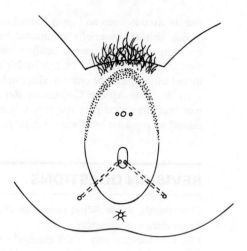

Fig. 5.4 Infibulation – anterior two-thirds of labia majora also excised.

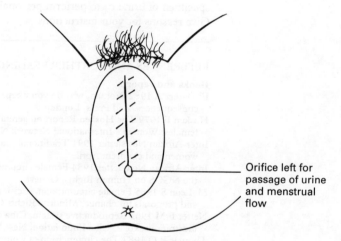

Fig. 5.5 Infibulated vulva showing 'suturing' with thorns as used in primitive society. Thorns are removed when remains of the labia have united.

Orifice left for passage of urine and menstrual flow

professional life, be responsible for the care of a circumcised lady during pregnancy, labour and the puerperium. Such a woman should be referred to the consultant obstetrician for if vaginal delivery is to be the method of choice, an anterior episiotomy at least, will most certainly be required if excision or infibulation has been performed. Suturing is a controversial issue and some obstetricians leave the wound to heal by granulation, since it will be ruptured again at subsequent deliveries. Caesarean section might be considered by some obstetricians but it is extremely important, for cultural reasons, that the decision be discussed with the husband as well as his wife. The failure to deliver her first baby vaginally can lead to her possible rejection as a 'real' woman and wife.

The World Health Organization, together with UNICEF, has assured governments that it will support national efforts to combat female circumcision and gives special attention to the training of all health visitors, especially traditional birth attendants. The WHO has consistently and unequivocally advised that female circumcision should not be practised by any health professionals in any setting, including hospitals or other health establishments.

At the Inter-African Committee Regional Conference in 1991 it was recommended that the terms 'female circumcision' and 'excision' be replaced by 'female genital mutilations'.

REVISION QUESTIONS

Describe the vulva. What pathological conditions of the vulva may occur during pregnancy?

Describe the anatomy of the external female genital organs.

Describe the anatomy of the external female genital organs. Of what importance is this knowledge a) to all women b) to a midwife.

Describe how you would instruct a patient a) to collect a midstream specimen of urine b) to perform personal vulval and perineal toilet. Give reasons for your instructions.

REFERENCES AND FURTHER READING

Books and reports
El Dareer A 1982 Woman, why do you weep? Circumcision and its consequences. Zed Press, London
Hosken F 1979 The Hosken Report on genital and sexual mutilation of females. Women's International Network News, Lexington, MA
Inter-African Newsletter 1991 Traditional practices affecting health of women and children. April
Inter-African Newsletter 1984 Female circumcision. Special Committee of the NGOS on Human Rights, Geneva
McLean S 1985 Female circumcision, excision and infibulation. The facts and proposals for change. Minority Rights Group, London
Netter F M 1965 Reproductive system. Ciba collection of medical illustrations, vol 2. Ciba Foundation, New York
Thomas R O 1987 The circumcision of women: a strategy for eradication. Zed Books, London

Articles
Lanjali M, Toubia N 1990 Female circumcision. IPPF Medical Bulletin 24: 1–2
Lightfoot R, Shan E 1990 Special needs of ritually circumcised women patients. Journal of Obstetric, Gynecological and Neonatal Nursing 20(2): 102–107
Livingstone A 1991 A continuing problem in Britain. British Medical Journal 302: 497–498

6 The vagina

(Plate 2A and B, Plate 3A)

Situation The vagina is a potential canal which extends from the vulva to the uterus. It runs upwards and backwards parallel to the plane of the pelvic brim. It is surrounded and supported by the pelvic floor muscles.

Shape Its shape is that of a potential tube, the walls normally lying in close contact with each other but becoming easily separated.

Size Because the cervix enters the vagina at right angles, the posterior vaginal wall is longer than the anterior wall when the uterus is anteverted. The anterior wall is approximately 7.5 cm long and the posterior wall 11.5 cm long. Should the uterus be retroverted, then these measurements will be reversed.

Gross structure **Four fornices** are formed where the cervix projects into the vagina. These are named **anterior**, **posterior**, or **lateral** according to their position; the posterior fornix is the largest. At the external orifice of the vagina, the **hymen** covers the opening or, if the hymen has been ruptured, the **carunculae myrtiformes** are found instead.

Microscopic structure 1. *Squamous epithelium* is a type of modified skin and forms the vaginal lining
2. *Vascular connective tissue*
3. *Muscle coat* is arranged in two layers of involuntary muscle fibres:
   a. inner circular fibres
   b. outer longitudinal fibres
   Although this muscle coat is rather thin, it is nevertheless very strong
4. *Fascia* is made up of loose connective tissue which is part of the pelvic cellular tissue

The walls of the vagina do not lie smoothly but fall into transverse folds, **the rugae**, which allow for distension. In a patient who has borne several children the rugae have been stretched several times, and are therefore not so obvious on inspection.

Blood supply Vaginal and uterine arteries, branches of the internal iliac artery, form a plexus round the vagina.
Venous drainage is by corresponding vessels.

Lymphatic drainage Drainage of the lower third of the vagina is into the inguinal glands, while the upper two thirds is into the internal and external iliac glands.

Nerve supply   Sympathetic and parasympathetic nerves from the Lee-Frankenhäuser (sacral) plexus serve that portion of the vagina which lies above the levatores ani muscles. The pudendal nerve supplies the lower vaginal area.

Relations (Fig. 6.1)   *Anterior*: Base of bladder rests on upper half of vagina. The urethra is embedded in lower half
Posterior: (a) pouch of Douglas – superiorly, (b) rectum – centrally, (c) perineal body – inferiorly
Lateral: Pubococcygeus muscle below. Pelvic fascia containing ureter above
Inferior: Structures of the vulva
Superior: Cervix

Functions   • Entrance for spermatozoa
• Exit for menstrual flow and products of conception
• Helps to support the uterus
• Helps to prevent infection

There is an acid medium in the vagina provided by **Doederlein's bacilli** which are normal inhabitants there. They act on the glycogen in the vaginal walls and convert it to lactic acid. The amount of glycogen in the vaginal walls is under the cyclical influence of ovarian hormones and therefore tends to vary – especially with the onset of pregnancy. The normal pH of vaginal fluid varies between 3.8 and 4.5.

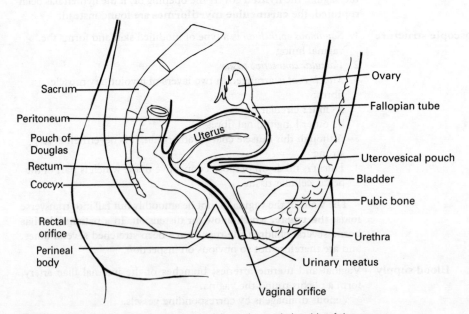

Fig. 6.1   Cross-section through female pelvis to show relationship of the organs.

The acid medium destroys pathogenic organisms but if the bacilli are absent or reduced in number the acidity of the vagina is altered, resulting in a consequent vaginitis.

Expectant mothers should therefore be advised not to use anti-septic preparations in the bath or for vulval or vaginal toilet purposes except under medical supervision.

VAGINAL DISCHARGES AND SEXUALLY-TRANSMITTED DISEASES IN RELATION TO PREGNANCY

Physiological A clear, inoffensive discharge, just a little heavier than usual, is quite normal during pregnancy and is brought about by the extra hormonal activity. No treatment is necessary except for advising more frequent vulval hygiene and changes of underclothing.

Blood If blood is passed per vaginam at any stage of pregnancy, the patient should seek medical advice at once. Early in pregnancy it may signify an impending abortion and, after the 28th week, it is a possible sign of early placental separation. It is important that the actual cause be found as soon as possible, as the life of both mother and baby may be in danger.

Moniliasis

Causative organism is a fungus, *Candida albicans*, which thrives in a more acid medium. It is therefore often found in association with pregnancy as well as in diabetes.

Signs and symptoms White curdy patches can be seen on the vaginal walls and there is a greyish-white staining of vulval pads and underclothes. There is associated vulval and vaginal irritation.

Diagnosis is easy as the clinical appearance is distinctive, but a high vaginal swab should always be sent to the laboratory to confirm that *Candida albicans* is present.

Treatment is usually a course of **nystatin** vaginal pessaries. One pessary, which contains 100 000 units, is inserted nightly for 14 nights.

Alternatively **clotrimazole** vaginal pessaries 100 mg are inserted nightly for 14 nights.

Should the infection be transmitted to the fetus during delivery, a troublesome 'thrush' and/or eye infection develops. It is therefore essential that the mother's infection be cleared before delivery is imminent. The infected infant will require oral nystatin or eye-drops as prescribed by the paediatrician.

Trichomoniasis

Causative organism is the protozoon *Trichomonas vaginalis*.

Signs and symptoms A profuse, greenish-yellow, watery, frothy discharge with a distinctive stale, offensive odour is present. The patient complains

Table 6.1   Vaginal discharge and sexually transmitted diseases

	Moniliasis	Trichomoniasis	Gonorrhoea	NSGI Chlamydia	Herpes genitalis	Syphilis	AIDS
Causative organism	Candida albican (yeast fungus)	Trichomona vaginalis (protozoon)	Neisseria gonorrhoeae (bacillus)	Chlamydia trachomatis (parasite)	Herpes simplex Type II (virus)	Treponema pallidum (spirochaete)	AIDS virus – Human immuno-deficiency virus (HIV)
Incubation period			3–10 days following sexual intercourse (infected partner)			9–90 days	Variable HIV antibodies present in blood 3 months after infection
S & S	Inflammation and irritation of vagina & vulva White curdy patches on vaginal walls Grey staining of vulval pads or underclothes	Profuse greenish yellow frothy vaginal discharge Inflammation and irritation of vulval & vagina	Sometimes none Greenish offensive puslike vaginal discharge Inflammation of genital Urethritis Dysuria	Mucopurulent vaginal discharge Dysuria Cervicitis	Stinging, tingling, irritation in affected area of vesicles (genital & anal areas, sometimes mouth) Flu-like symptoms Enlarged lymph nodes	Three stages: 1. Primary chancre and enlarged lymph glands 2. Flu like symptoms Condylomata 3. 2–10 years later Gummata affecting body organs, bones, nerves etc.	Early signs: Akin to glandular fever Then: Diminishing resistance to infection as disease progresses: PGL ARC AIDS
Diagnosis	Culture of organism Found on microscopy & examination of HVS in lab	Culture of organism Found on microscopy & examination of HVS in lab	Culture of swabs in path. lab	Culture of organism vaginal swab in path. lab	Virology studies in path. lab	Serological test Positive 3 weeks after infection FTA & TPI tests	Only made on request Serological
Treatment	Nystatin vaginal pessaries 100 000 units nightly for 14 nights	Oral metronidazole 200 µm Penotrate vaginal pessaries 5 µm	Crystalline penicillin 5 megaunits i.m.i. Probenecid 1g	Erythromycin 500 µm b.d. 14–21 days	Analgesics Ice packs Saline sitz baths Acyclovir	i.m.i. procaine penicillin 600 000 units daily 7–14 days	Zidovudine Interferons Soluble CD4 Pentamidine Acyclovir Immunovira IZAT

of acute irritation and inflammation of the vulva and vagina, which look very red and sore. There is increased frequency of micturition, dysuria and dyspareunia.

Diagnosis   is confirmed by the laboratory when a high vaginal swab is cultured. As the condition is associated with gonorrhoea, the latter condition must be excluded and the swab must be examined for *Neisseria gonorrhoeae*.

Treatment   is the administration of oral **metronidazole** 200 mg, usually given daily for 10 days, but its use is better avoided in early pregnancy because there is still some concern regarding its potential teratogenic effects. Penotrane vaginal pessaries 5 mg may be used to relieve some of the discomfort.

This infection is also likely to be transmitted to the sexual partner, who should be counselled and treated accordingly.

Gonorrhoea

Causative organism is *Neisseria gonorrhoeae*, a bacterium also known as the **gonococcus**.

Incubation period is 3–10 days. 50% of patients are symptom-free following the incubation period, so that where the woman has more than one sexual partner the disease can be spread very rapidly.

Signs and symptoms The symptomatic patient complains of a greenish-coloured, offensive, pus-like discharge which causes the genital area to be inflamed and oedematous. It is accompanied by urethritis and dysuria and it is possible to milk pus from Skene's tubules. A Bartholin's abscess may be present. About 50% of infected patients have an associated trichomonal infection.

Diagnosis is made by culture of swabs which are taken from the vagina and cervix, the urethra, the rectum and the mouth. An intravenous sample of blood is tested to exclude syphilis.

Treatment Crystalline penicillin 5 megaunits with lignocaine is given by intramuscular injection. Probenecid 1 g is given to obtain slow excretion of the antibiotic.

Three examinations are carried out at weekly intervals to assess this patient's progress.

All her sexual partners should be traced in order that they may receive treatment.

Gonococcal infection transmitted to the infant during delivery can result in **ophthalmia neonatorum** which is a notifiable disease. It can result in blindness. The infant must be isolated. Penicillin eye drops are administered in a course of intensive therapy and systemic penicillin is administered according to the baby's weight. All contaminated articles are a potential source of infection and should be incinerated wherever possible. If gonorrhoea is untreated in early pregnancy, the patient may abort or the baby be stillborn.

The infection is likely to spread throughout the genital tract causing a generalised pelvic infection and possible future infertility.

Non-specific genital infection (*Chlamydia*)

Causative organism is Chlamydia trachomatis, a small, parasitic unicellular organism.

Signs and symptoms The vaginal discharge is mucopurulent. Cervicitis and pelvic inflammatory disease often recur as a consequence of the infection. The patient complains of dysuria. History-taking may elicit that the woman's sexual partner has been, or is being, treated for non-specific urethritis.

Diagnosis   is made when the laboratory detects *Chlamydia trachomatis* in vaginal smears.

Treatment   Erythromycin 500 mg is given twice daily for 14–21 days.

Tetracycline therapy is used if the condition is not associated with pregnancy.

If the condition remains untreated, it will give rise to general pelvic infection and infertility. If the infection is transmitted to the infant, there is the danger of neonatal eye infections, and of neonatal pneumonia.

It seems logical at this stage in the text to include other sexually transmitted diseases, although the following conditions are not associated with vaginal discharge:

Syphilis

Causative organism   is a spirochaete, *Treponema pallidum*, and the incubation period is between 9 and 90 days.

Signs and symptoms   These occur at three intervals:

Primary stage

The initial lesion of syphilis is a chancre which appears at the site of infection. 95% of chancres appear on the genitalia but they are sometimes seen on the lips or the nipple. A chancre is a hard raised area about the size of a 20 p piece. It is painless, often unnoticed and heals in less than 8 weeks. Occasionally there is an area of oedema around the chancre. Where oedema of only one labium is apparent, the possibility of syphilitic chancre on its inner surface should not be disregarded, and a full inspection should be made with a gloved hand.

The lymphatic glands in the vicinity of the chancre are enlarged, i.e.:

- the inguinal glands on the corresponding side if there is a genital chancre
- the axillary glands on the corresponding side if there is a chancre on the nipple
- the parotid glands if there is a chancre on the upper lip.

The glands are hard, feel like almonds, are painless and do not suppurate. During this stage, the infected person is highly infectious; the discharge from the chancre being the source of infection.

Serological tests are not positive until at least 3 weeks following the infection.

Secondary stage

The infected person complains of headache, sore throat, hoarseness and general malaise. There is aching of the bones and joints, skin rashes have become evident and mild pyrexia is present. Condylomata, soft wart-like growths, develop around the anus and on the vulva. This stage continues to be symptomatic for 3–12 months and then passes into a latent period.

Tertiary stage

This is rarely seen today in a civilisation where there is adequate publicity about, and provision for, treating venereal infections in confidence.

When syphilis is untreated, it may be 2–3 years before further manifestation of symptoms occurs. Small swellings, gummata, occur in any organ or body structure that is attacked by the spirochaetes. These swellings are really a defence mechanism, being made up of debris and fibrous tissue, but their presence causes pressure, and therefore trauma, to surrounding tissues. As a consequence, bones may fracture or body organs cease to function properly. Late complications involve the cardiovascular system, the central nervous system (general paralysis of the insane), or the spinal cord may be involved, resulting in locomotor ataxia.

Syphilis tends to be latent in pregnancy and there are usually no presenting signs or symptoms unless the infection has occurred following conception.

Diagnosis All pregnant women have serological tests for syphilis and these include:

- *Fluorescent treponemal antibody test* (FTA): an easy, quick and specific test
- Treponema pallidum *immobilisation test* (TPI): a specific test, but it takes longer to perform.

If these tests are positive, then the pregnant woman requires treatment and her sexual partners should be traced by a venereal disease social worker and treated as necessary.

Treatment Intramuscular injection (i.m.i.) of procaine penicillin 600 000 units daily for 7–14 days.

Further serological tests are carried out over a 2-year period. The woman will be contacted by a venereal disease social worker. All sexual partners should be contacted too, and referred to the special clinic for treatment.

Obstetric significance

As already stated, syphilis is usually latent in pregnancy and is diagnosed as the result of routine haematology. If infective lesions are present, then the midwife must protect herself from infection by wearing a gown and gloves and must ensure their safe disposal. If treatment is begun before the 20th week of pregnancy, then prognosis is good and the mother can be considered as being non-infectious 48 hours after commencing penicillin therapy. In most instances the infant will be born symptom-free, but he cannot be regarded as being syphilis-free until serological tests have been carried out when he is 6 weeks old, because a sample of cord blood is likely to contain antibodies from his treated mother. He is therefore treated with i.m.i. procaine penicillin according to his birthweight and isolated for his first 48 hours.

Should the mother book late at the antenatal clinic or be admitted in labour untreated, the outlook is unhappy. **Intrauterine infection** and **late abortion** or **intrauterine death**, often with a **macerated fetus**, are the likely outcome. The **placenta is large, pale and unhealthy-looking**. An untreated mother means a congenitally syphilitic infant and if born alive he may soon show the small blisters on his hands and feet of **pemphigus neonatorum** (a notifiable disease). Within the first year his nasal bones begin to necrose, giving the typical **saddle-nose** of syphilis. This infant is therefore treated with i.m.i. procaine penicillin 150 000 units daily for 10 days and a second course is given 1 month later if his blood tests are still positive.

Herpes genitalis

Causative organism   The herpes simplex virus, usually Type 2.

Herpes simplex virus Type 1 causes sores around the mouth and nose and, more rarely, in the eyes or in the genital and anal areas.

Herpes simplex virus Type 2 causes sores in the genital and anal areas and, more rarely, in the mouth.

Incubation period   3–10 days.

Mode of infection   There may be some degree of self-infection. By touching a sore on the mouth, the finger may transmit the virus to the genital region. Infection may also occur as the result of oral sex.

Signs and symptoms   Stinging, tingling or itching sensations are felt in the genital and/or oral areas. Where nerve fibres are affected, the virus travels up the nerve to its root and remains there. There is mild pyrexia, a feeling of general malaise, headache, backache and flu-like symptoms. Back pain may extend to the thighs and the legs. Small vesicles form in affected areas but these will obviously not be visible if they occur in the vagina or rectum. The blisters rupture, leaving small red lesions which are painful and take about 7 days to heal. Dysuria occurs but this is not associated with increased frequency of micturition. Inguinal lymph nodes are enlarged and painful. The primary attack lasts between 6 and 122 days and may then be re-activated again and again.

Diagnosis   Virology studies are made by the pathological laboratory.

Treatment
- Analgesics and ice packs may be used to relieve pain
- Sitz baths using a saline solution may be taken three times daily
- The sores should be kept as dry as possible. Application of witch hazel is sometimes helpful in relieving pain
- Sexual intercourse should be avoided.

Obstetric significance

1. *If intrauterine infection occurs* it can result in:
   - Intrauterine death
   - Premature labour
   - Neonatal encephalitis or other virus infection

   There is a high fetal mortality rate
2. *If membranes rupture*, an antiherpes drug, **acyclovir**, is given to the mother
3. *Elective caesarean section* is the safest method of delivery for the infant
4. *Immunoglobulin* is given to the infant after delivery

Autoimmune deficiency syndrome (AIDS)

Causative organism

The AIDS virus HIV I or II (Human immunodeficiency virus)

Those at risk include homosexuals (who could also infect their female partners), drug addicts, those who take casual sexual partners and those who require blood transfusions in areas where blood donors are not screened. There has been a risk for patients receiving artificial insemination by donor treatment.

Signs and symptoms

These are vague at first and akin to glandular fever. Later in the disease, the immune system is badly damaged and there is a diminishing resistance to infection. Conditions that may develop include ***Pneumocystis carinii* pneumonia, Kaposi's sarcoma.**

Diagnosis

is made only on request. Those who are discovered to be seropositive or who have developed AIDS will need supportive counselling and assistance.

Treatment

There is no satisfactory treatment to date. Emphasis must therefore lie in prevention. Education of the general public is the best means of prevention. Known sufferers may be prescribed the following:

- Drugs which attack the virus HPA 23
- Drugs which stimulate the immune system – Immunovira IZAT.

Obstetric significance

The AIDS virus can cross the placental membrane and may cause intrauterine growth retardation or microcephaly.

All blood loss and breast milk transmit the virus and are possible sources of infection.

All precautions as for prevention of transmitting hepatitis B are used during delivery.

VAGINAL EXAMINATION

Antenatal

At the woman's first visit to the antenatal clinic, the doctor working in remote areas where obstetric services are very limited will probably perform a vaginal examination for the following reasons:

- To confirm pregnancy
- To exclude abnormality of the pelvic organs
- To exclude abnormality of the bony pelvis.

A further examination is often made at about the 36th week of pregnancy:

- To exclude later abnormalities of the pelvic organs
- To assess the size of the pelvis in relation to the fetal head and to ensure that the head is able to pass through the pelvic brim
- To ensure that the pelvic outlet is adequate.

In countries where adequate obstetric facilities are available and modern technology is standard practice, these examinations are no longer necessary or advocated.

In labour

The midwife may perform vaginal examinations during labour **unless**:

- The woman has a history of antepartum haemorrhage
- She has been admitted for 'trial of labour'
- Labour is any way not proceeding satisfactorily.

Indications for vaginal examination
- To determine the onset of labour
- To determine the presentation or engagement, if there is any doubt
- To exclude cord prolapse when membranes rupture early
- To determine dilatation of the cervix before giving rectal suppositories
- To determine dilatation of the cervix before giving analgesic drugs
- To confirm full dilatation of the cervix when there is any doubt.

Technique
1. Explain the procedure to the mother
2. Ask her to empty her bladder
3. Examine the abdomen by
   a. Inspection
   b. Palpation
   c. Auscultation
4. Vulval toilet is performed, the right hand being kept clean
5. Index and middle finger of right hand are used to make the examination.

NB To perform a vaginal examination without first carrying out an abdominal palpation might be compared to a blind man looking in a dark room for a black cat.

If, on abdominal palpation, the fetal back is palpated to the right and is lying anteriorly in the abdomen, and if this is confirmed by hearing the fetal heart at maximum intensity mid-way between the umbilicus and the right anterior superior iliac spine, then the midwife will know where, on vaginal examination, the landmarks on the fetal skull should be. If fetal landmarks are not where she expects to find then she will need to ask herself why – and perhaps ask for a second opinion.

Observations to record

External genitalia	Oedema, varicose veins, warts, perineal scars.
Condition of vagina	It should feel warm and be easily distended with the fingers. A hot, dry vagina indicates a raised temperature. A tight vagina indicates a tense patient. Any vaginal discharge is noted.
Cervix	Note whether the cervix is effaced, whether soft or rigid, whether the presenting part is well applied to it or whether there is an anterior or posterior lip.
Dilatation of the os	usually assessed by the number of fingerbreadths that the os will admit, i.e. one finger = 2 cm.
Membranes	Record whether there are any bulging, intact or ruptured. If ruptured, the colour of the liquor should be noted.
Presentation	1. Ensure that the head is presenting or identify the presenting part 2. Assess whether it is above or below or at the level of the ischial spines 3. Confirm position by finding sutures and fontanelles and relating them to the maternal pelvis (Fig. 6.2) 4. Note the degree of moulding or caput formation.
Pelvic outlet	The ischial spines should be palpated and the size of the pubic arch should be estimated.

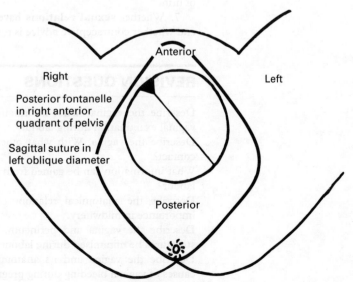

Anterior

Right

Left

Posterior fontanelle in right anterior quadrant of pelvis

Sagittal suture in left oblique diameter

Posterior

Fig. 6.2 Vaginal examination. Right occipito anterior position of fetus.

When the fingers are withdrawn from the vagina, they should be examined for meconium staining. These observations should be recorded on the mother's notes and illustrated with a diagram (Fig. 6.2).

Rectum   During the examination a full rectum will be easily identified.

If more than one vaginal examination needs to be performed during the course of labour, it is essential to relate to the latest data from preceding examinations, particularly in respect of:

- Descent and flexion of the fetal head
- Dilatation of the cervix
- Presence and/or oedema of a lip of cervix
- Colour of amniotic fluid.

Postnatal

6 weeks following delivery the mother is seen at the postnatal clinic to check her general health and well-being (see Chs 2, 3, 7, 8). A vaginal examination is carried out as part of this general examination and the doctor will note:

1. That the **uterus** is anteverted, anteflexed and of normal size
2. That the **cervix** has re-formed and that the **external os** is only a slit-like aperture
3. That the **cervix** is healthy. It is examined using a light and a speculum to exclude cervical erosions. A cervical smear is sent to the cytology technician unless one was taken during pregnancy.
4. That all vaginal and perineal **lacerations** have healed
5. The tone of the **pelvic floor muscles**
6. Whether any degree of urinary or faecal **incontinence** is present and if there is stress urgency, dysuria or increased frequency of urine
7. Whether **sexual relations** have been resumed satisfactorily and whether contraceptive advice is required.

REVISION QUESTIONS

Describe the vagina. What information may be obtained from a vaginal examination during labour?

Describe the vagina. With what other structures does it come in contact?

What information can be gained from a vaginal examination during labour?

Describe the anatomical relations of the vagina. Indicate their importance in midwifery.

Describe the vagina and perineum. How may injuries to these structures be minimised during labour and delivery?

Describe the vagina and its anatomical relations. What are the causes of vaginal bleeding during pregnancy?

List the indications for vaginal examination (a) in pregnancy, (b) at the postnatal examination.

How can a midwife identify the different types of vaginal discharges in pregnancy? Give the treatment for each condition.

List the indications for vaginal examination in labour. What information can the midwife obtain from this examination?

Describe in detail how a midwife may assess the progress of labour (a) by abdominal examination, (b) by vaginal examination.

Describe the anatomy of the vagina. Discuss the relevance of the information a midwife may obtain when performing a vaginal examination during labour.

Write short notes on:

AIDS
Chlamydia
Gonorrhoea
Moniliasis
Trichomoniasis
Syphilitic chancre
Serological tests in syphilis.

REFERENCES AND FURTHER READING

Books and reports
Adler M W 1990 ABC of sexually transmitted diseases, 2nd edn. British Medical Association, London
Collier C 1987 The 20th century plague. Lion, Tring
Dixon P 1987 The truth about AIDS. Kingsway, Eastbourne
Gillespie O 1983 Herpes: what to do when you have it. Sheldon, London
Terrence Higgins Trust 1990 HIV and AIDS: information for women. Terrence Higgins Trust, London
Terrence Higgins Trust Medical Group 1991 AIDS and HIV: medical briefing. Terrence Higgins Trust, London
Llewellyn Jones D 1985 Herpes, AIDS and other sexually transmitted diseases. Faber & Faber, London
Thin R N 1982 Lecture notes on sexually transmitted diseases. Blackwell Scientific Publications, Oxford

Articles
Brierley J 1987 Immunodeficiency virus: the challenge of a lifetime. Midwives' Chronicle 100: x–xiii
Parker D 1989 Sexually transmitted diseases and pregnancy. Midwife, Health Visitor and Community Nurse 25(5): 194–198

Help lines
Body Positive Women's Group 071-490-1225
British Pregnancy Advisory Service 0564-793-225
Brook Advisory Centre 071-703-9660
Drugs Alcohol Women Now 071-700-4653
Family Planning Association 071-636-7866
National AIDS Helpline 0800-567-123
Positively Women 071-490-5515
Terrence Higgins Trust 071-242-1010
Women's Health and Reproductive Rights Information Centre 071-251-6560

7 The cervix

Although the cervix is part of the uterus, its structure and function differ from the main body of the uterus and it is therefore described separately.

Situation It forms the lower third of the uterus and is the area below the isthmus which includes the internal and external os. It enters the vagina at right angles and is sometimes called the 'neck' of the uterus.

Shape The cervical canal is fusiform and the cervix as a whole tends to be barrel-shaped.

Size In adult life the cervix is 2.5 cm long and, as stated, forms one-third of the total length of the uterus. During intrauterine life, however, it forms the greater part of the uterus and then in the last weeks of pregnancy there is an accelerated growth of the uterine body brought about by the high levels of maternal oestrogenic hormones. At the time of birth, the cervix and body of the uterus are approximately equal in size. When the ovarian hormones are activated at puberty there is a further acceleration of uterine body growth until it is approximately twice the length of the cervix. The diagnosis of an infantile uterus in an adult woman is made partly by assessing these relative proportions.

Gross structure (Fig. 7.1)

The supravaginal cervix is that portion of the cervix which lies outside and above the vagina. Superiorly, it meets the border of the uterus at the **isthmus**.

The infravaginal cervix is that portion which projects into the vagina.

The internal os opens into the cavity of the uterus. Although not a sphincter in the true sense of the word, it dilates during labour. Incompetence of the cervix at this level results in spontaneous abortion in the mid-trimester of pregnancy. Incompetence is sometimes due to a congenital anomaly, sometimes associated with dilatation of the cervix during a dilatation and curettage operation, and is particularly associated with the surgical termination of pregnancy in young primigravidae. It is also sometimes associated with a large cone biopsy carried out when abnormal cervical cells have been found on cytological examination.

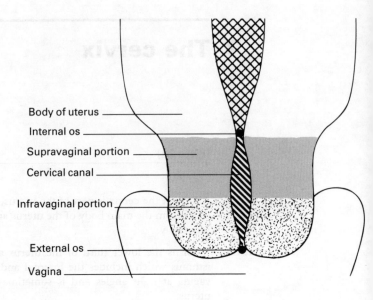

Body of uterus

Internal os

Supravaginal portion

Cervical canal

Infravaginal portion

External os

Vagina

Fig. 7.1 Gross structure of the cervix.

The external os opens into the vagina at the lower end of the cervical canal. On pelvic examination it is found at the level of the upper border of the symphysis pubis. In the multiparous woman it is recognised on vaginal examination by being circular in shape, smooth and with a dimple in the centre. After the 36th week of pregnancy, the 'dimple' will admit a finger tip. In the multigravida it is a transverse, slit-like aperture with an irregular edge and will easily admit a finger tip even in early pregnancy. It is known as a **'multip's os'**.

The cervical canal lies between the internal and external os.

Microscopic structure There are three layers of tissue.

Endometrium is the inner layer. It contains many racemose glands, some of which are ciliated to facilitate the passage of spermatozoa. The tissue is arranged in folds, the **arbor vitae**, the folds allowing dilatation of the cervix to occur without trauma. In the multigravid patient, the arbor vitae becomes flattened out with successive pregnancies. The cervical endometrium is more glandular than that in the main body of the uterus and it is not shed during menstruation. Nevertheless it is affected by oestrogenic hormones and at the time of ovulation there is an increase in the glandular secretion, which also becomes less viscous.

Muscle Involuntary muscle fibres are mingled with dense collagenous tissue which gives the cervix a fibrous nature. It is not possible to state relative proportions of each, since this appears to be dependent upon the hormone levels of each individual woman. The 'average' muscle content is said to be about 10%. Longitudinal muscle fibres from the uterus pass into the cervix but there is a preponderance of spiral fibres which run in both clockwise and anticlockwise directions and lie in circular formation in the cervix.

Although the amount of muscle fibre in the uterine body is increased considerably during pregnancy, histological studies show that there is a negligible increase in the cervix.

Peritoneum covers that part of the cervix which lies above the vagina. It is loosely applied in the area where it reflects up and over the bladder. This allows both the bladder and uterus to modify their positions as required.

The infravaginal cervix has an outer coat of stratified epithelium which is continuous with that of the vaginal lining. It continues a short distance into the cervical canal to meet the cervical endometrium at the **squamocolumnar junction** – the commonest site of cervical cancer.

Blood supply The blood is supplied through the uterine arteries, and venous drainage is through the uterine veins.

Lymphatic drainage The lymphatic drainage is into the internal iliac and sacral glands.

Nerve supply Sympathetic and parasympathetic nerves from the Lee–Frankenhäuser (sacral) plexus provide the nerve supply.

Supports

Transverse cervical ligaments extend from the cervix to the lateral walls of the pelvis.

Pubocervical ligaments run forwards from the cervix to the pubic bones.

Uterosacral ligaments extend from the cervix and pass backwards to the sacrum.

Functions
- It helps to *prevent infection* entering the uterus
- It dilates and withdraws during labour to *enable vaginal delivery of the fetus and placenta*
- Following delivery, the cervix returns almost to its non-pregnant state.

Relations *Anterior*: the uterovesical pouch of peritoneum and the bladder
Posterior: the pouch of Douglas and the rectum
Lateral: the broad ligament and the ureters, which are crossed by the uterine arteries

The foregoing description is of the non-pregnant cervix. Certain changes occur during pregnancy, labour and the puerperium.

The cervix and pregnancy The blood supply to the cervix is increased during pregnancy so that it becomes softer and more blue in colour. The cervical glands secrete more mucus and a plug of this mucoid material, the **operculum**, fills the cervical canal. Its main function is to close it and thus minimise the risk of ascending genital tract infection. The cervical endometrium does not undergo decidual changes in pregnancy like uterine endometrium.

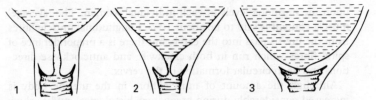

Fig. 7.2 Changes in the cervix of a primiparous patient: (1) before labour (2) cervix being taken up (3) cervix fully effaced.

Towards the end of pregnancy rising levels of the hormone **relaxin** effect softening of the collagenous content of the cervix.

During the last 2 weeks of pregnancy the cervical canal of the primigravida is taken up into the lower uterine segment when engagement of the fetal head exerts downwards pressure on the cervical tissues around the internal os.

The cervical canal is then no longer fusiform in shape but becomes funnel-shaped, the wide part of the funnel being at the level of the internal os. Immediately prior to the onset of labour the external os barely admits a finger tip but the canal has been reduced to at least half its length.

In this state the cervix of the primigravida is said to be 'ripe' (Fig. 7.2).

In the multigravid patient whose abdominal muscles lack the firm tone of the primigravida, the fetal head does not engage until labour is established. As there is no pressure on the cervix, there is therefore no effacement until the fetal head has descended. Effacement and dilation of the cervix then occur simultaneously once labour is established (Fig. 7.3).

Complications of pregnancy

Cervical erosions are believed to be of hormonal origin and are normally left untreated. They often cause a little blood loss but usually clear spontaneously.

Cervical polyps are diagnosed only by inspection on vaginal examination when they cause a small blood loss. No treatment is carried out during pregnancy.

Congenital abnormalities are occasionally discovered for the first time at a vaginal examination during pregnancy.

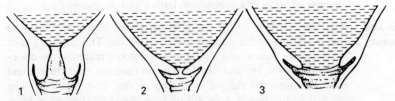

Fig. 7.3 Changes in the cervix of a multiparous patient: (1) before labour (2) cervix being taken up (3) cervix fully effaced.

Carcinoma of the cervix is very rarely associated with pregnancy but, if it is diagnosed, treatment depends largely upon how advanced the disease is and at what stage of pregnancy it is diagnosed. Further details will be found later in this chapter.

Incompetent cervix The more usual causes of cervical incompetence have already been described but it may also be caused by trauma during a difficult delivery, e.g. severe lacerations or annular detachment of the cervix. Whatever the cause, at some time between the 12th and 28th week of pregnancy, as intrauterine pressure starts to increase, the cervix dilates, the membranes rupture and the fetus is expelled.

Where there is a history of repeated abortion caused by an incompetent cervix, the **Shirodkar operation** is carried out. The usual time for the procedure is at the 14th week of pregnancy but it is occasionally performed before pregnancy has actually commenced. A purse-string suture of tape is inserted as high as possible around the cervix, sometimes, but not always, without incising the epithelial tissue. The suture must, of course, be removed at the 38th week of pregnancy or at the onset of labour – whichever occurs first. If not removed, there will be severe cervical trauma as labour progresses and the cervix tries to dilate. If delivery is to be by caesarean section, then the suture is removed immediately prior to surgery.

The cervix in labour Ripening of the cervix towards the end of pregnancy has been described on page 108.

Effacement It has just been explained that, in the primigravida, effacement of the cervix commences in the last weeks of pregnancy. It is completed during the first stage of labour, and once completely effaced, the external os commences to dilate. In the multigravida it is more common for the fetal head not to engage until labour is established and so it is not applied to the cervix until that time. (Fig. 7.3) Effacement and dilatation of the cervical os in the multigravida then occur simultaneously once labour has commenced.

Dilatation of the cervix The first stage of labour is defined as being the stage of cervical dilatation. It commences with uterine contractions which bring about dilatation of the external os and is completed when the cervix has opened widely enough to allow the fetal head to pass through.

'Taking up' or withdrawal of the cervix is accomplished as the longitudinal muscle fibres extending into the cervix from the body of the uterus contract and retract. The length of the cervix is thereby reduced and as it 'takes up' it becomes thinner as it merges into the lower uterine segment. When fully taken up (i.e. effaced), only a thin rim of cervix can be felt around the fetal head and there is no longer a cervical canal.

Once the cervix has been fully taken up, the external os continues to dilate until it has opened widely enough for the head to pass through. No cervix can be palpated at this time since the cervix has now been pulled upwards right over the fetal head.

It is possible for the midwife to assess the degree of effacement of the cervix and dilatation of the os by vaginal examination (see p. 100).

The cervix following delivery

The cervix **begins to close** and return to its non-pregnant state immediately after delivery. At the postnatal examination 6 weeks after the birth of the baby the cervix should have **re-formed** with an internal and external os and the cervical canal between them. The external os never again completely closes but becomes a slit-like aperture which is large enough to admit a finger tip. This is the **'multip's os.'**

Cervical erosions sometimes occur in association with pregnancy and give rise to an excessive and uncomfortable vaginal discharge. Because the causative factor is thought to be hormonal, treatment is rarely given during pregnancy. If such a lesion is present at the postnatal examination, it may of course have newly arisen following childbirth. In either instance a 6-week period is allowed to elapse during which time spontaneous healing may occur. If it has not healed, the woman should be referred to the gynaecology clinic. Laser treatment is carried out wherever the equipment is available. Otherwise the erosion is treated with cryosurgery or diathermy.

EARLY DIAGNOSIS OF CANCER OF THE CERVIX

Carcinoma of the cervix is beyond the scope of this book but because it is one of the commonest sites of cancer in women and because the midwife can play an effective role in screening sexually active women, it must be mentioned.

Incidence of carcinoma of the cervix – women at risk

Age

For many years women in the 35–55 age group were considered to be particularly at risk of cervical cancer but there has been an increase in the number of young women who have abnormal and even malignant cells diagnosed on cervical cytology. This ties in with the higher incidence of women who commence sexual activity at an early age, although they have not necessarily had many sexual partners. There have been girls of 16, presenting with venereal disease, who have also had pre-cancerous cells diagnosed at cervical screening and there is now considerable concern at the increasing incidence in this very young age group.

Promiscuity

This applies both to women and their sexual partners. There is a direct link between men with venereal disease (especially syphilis) and cervical cancer in their partners.

Occupation/socio-economic group

Two quite separate studies demonstrated the relationship between cancer of the cervix and the husband's occupation. The wives of manual labourers, for example, building-site workers, dock labourers, farm labourers and lorry drivers appear to be four times more likely to develop cancer of the cervix than the wives of white-collar workers, teachers, doctors etc.

Most of these former groups would be classified in the lower socio-economic groups where perhaps good standards of hygiene are not so easily attainable or recognised as being of such importance. Generally speaking, women in these lower socio-economic groups also tend to commence sexual activity at an earlier age.

It should also be borne in mind that, while class differences tend to be disappearing, promiscuity is increasing in all social groups. It is also recognised that there is a lowered incidence of cervical cancer in women whose husbands have been circumcised and that it is unknown in virgins.

Causative factors Having described the women particularly at risk, it should nevertheless be understood that all sexually active women are subject to some risk, even if they are faithful to their husbands. Some women may feel that to have a 'suspicious' diagnosis as the result of a cervical smear is likely to carry the same sort of stigma as venereal disease and these fears must be allayed.

It is now recognised that the herpes virus is associated with cervical cancer.

Men whose wives have developed the disease are known to have high histone levels in the coating of their sperm. These histones disrupt normal cell mechanisms and have the potential to induce the growth of tumours. The development of a vaccine and preventive treatment of all young girls before puberty is still to be developed. Work is also being carried out on trying to identify men with high histone levels. This theory, however, does not account for the low incidence of cervical cancer in those women whose husbands have been circumcised. Meanwhile, barrier methods of contraception are believed to reduce the risk of cervical cancer and their use can be suggested as a preventive measure.

Diagnosis All women who are sexually active should be screened regularly. Antenatal, postnatal and family planning clinics provide an excellent opportunity for testing to be carried out, but arrangements can also be made with a general practitioner, health centre or well-woman clinic. Patients who attend clinics where sexually-transmitted diseases are diagnosed and treated will automatically be screened there. Unfortunately it still appears that the majority of women who attend for screening are the partners of white-collar workers, the group least at risk. It is therefore important that at ante- and postnatal clinics the midwife should note when a woman last had a **cervical smear test**, or if she has had one at all. Where necessary, the doctor conducting the examination should be informed if the test is due to be carried out.

Cervical smear test
(Fig. 7.4)

Technique The woman is normally placed in the dorsal position and the cervix

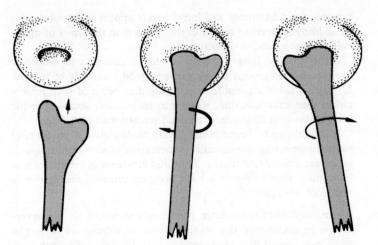

Fig. 7.4 Taking a cervical smear with an Ayre spatula.

is exposed with a Cusco speculum and inspected using a good light. An Ayre's spatula is used to scrape cells from around the external os and the squamocolumnar junction. One end of this spatula is more suitable for nullipara; the other end is larger and more suitable to take cells from the multip's os. The secretions are then smeared thinly on to a prepared, named glass slide and fixed.

Delay in 'fixing' may cause distortion of the cells.

If they are spread too thickly, the cells are difficult to examine under the microscope.

The smear is sent to the laboratory to be examined by an experienced technician who needs frequent and adequate breaks if his readings are to be accurate. This work demands a very high level of concentration.

Processing   All cells can be defined by microscopic examination according to the tissue from which they are derived. Cells of the female genital tract are more complicated in that they differ according to a woman's age, the phase of her menstrual cycle, any hormone therapy such as the contraceptive 'pill' and, of course, changes occurring in the antenatal and postnatal periods. Nevertheless, when cells are malignant, in addition to dysplasia, their nuclei and chromosome patterns are abnormal.

Where cells look 'suspicious' or are almost certainly malignant, they are reviewed by a consultant pathologist for confirmation before a report is issued to the general practitioner.

Follow-up   Women whose cells are quite normal should be informed of this and, if they are under 35 years of age, told that a reminder will be issued in about 5 years time when they will be due to report for a further test. Women over 35 years old should be tested at 3-yearly intervals.

If cells are 'suspicious' or almost certainly malignant, the woman is asked to attend the clinic for colposcopy, a special technique in which the cervix is examined with a microscope and a biopsy is taken for histology. In some instances laser therapy will be carried out simultaneously.

Further treatment   Following colposcopy, cytology and histology the consultant decides on one of the following treatments:

1. *Laser therapy* can be carried out in the outpatient department. The laser is used in conjunction with the colposcope and the abnormal cells are vaporised. The area heals quickly, leaving no fibrous tissue. This is suitable for carcinoma-in-situ, sometimes described as Stage 0.

2. *Cautery or diathermy*: Used where there is no access to a laser.

3. *Cone biopsy* is used of necessity if the abnormal cells are in, or extend up into, the cervical canal or if there is any suspicion of early invasive change. A cone-shaped excision of all the abnormal tissue is made and the patient is then asked to return to the clinic annually for further smear tests. A cone biopsy during pregnancy entails a risk of inducing an abortion. There is also the risk of haemorrhage from the pregnant vascular cervix. Where the cone biopsy is so extensive that it reaches the level of the internal os, there is the possible complication of the cervix being incompetent in any future pregnancies.

When abnormal cells of the cervix can be diagnosed before they become invasive and before any symptoms are produced, then carcinoma of the cervix becomes a preventable condition. But to be effective, treatment must be commenced at Stage 0, the stage of carcinoma-in-situ. The problem lies in reaching those women in the high-risk category who fail to attend screening clinics.

REVISION QUESTIONS

Describe the cervix uteri and the way in which it opens during the first stage of labour.

Describe the changes that take place in the cervix during pregnancy and normal labour.

Write short notes on:

Effacement and taking up of the cervix
Assessment of the cervix during the first stage of labour
Clinical evidence of full dilatation of the cervix
Incompetent cervix
Cervical cytology
Colposcopy
Shirodkar suture
Arbor vitae
Operculum
Multip's os
Cervical erosion

REFERENCES AND FURTHER READING

Books and reports

Jordan J, Singer A 1976 The cervix. W B Saunders, Philadelphia

Kenny A 1985 Cancer of the cervix in young women. In: Studd J (ed) Progress in Obstetrics and Gynaecology 5. Churchill Livingstone, Edinburgh

Philpott R H 1976 Biodynamics of the cervix in pregnancy and labour. In: Jordan J, Singer A The cervix. W B Saunders, Philadelphia

Quilliam S 1989 Positive smear. Penguin, Harmondsworth

Articles

Calder A 1988 Cervical ripening: physiology and therapy. Journal of Obstetrics and Gynaecology (suppl): 52–56

Cooper W 1979 Joining up a jigsaw. Nursing Mirror 149: 28–29

Granstrom L et al 1989 Changes in the connective tissue of corpus and cervix uteri during pregnancy. Journal of Obstetrics and Gynaecology 96(10): 1198–1202

Jackson G, Pendleton H J, Nichol B, Wittmann B K 1984 Diagnostic ultrasound in the assessment of patients with incompetent cervix. British Journal of Obstetrics and Gynaecology 91(3): 232–236

Kane R 1986 The cervical stitch. The Miscarriage Association, Ossett, UK

Kiriwi R et al 1983 Determination of the elastic properties of the cervix. Journal of Obstetrics and Gynecology 71(4)

Mylotte M, Jordan J 1979 Beaming in on women. Nursing Mirror 149: 26–28

Taylor R W 1975 Cervical cytology. Nursing Mirror 141: 58–59

8 The uterus

Development   The early development of the cervix and its changing relative proportions to the body of the uterus have been described in the previous chapter. In about 60% of women the uterus has reached its adult stage of development by the age of 15 years, since there is an acceleration of growth even before the menstrual cycle is established. Because of its sudden increase in weight, as well as its elongation during the adolescent phase of development, the uterine body leans forwards from the isthmus, (its narrowest area) and bends over slightly at this junction with the cervix. Normally, therefore, it adopts an anteverted and anteflexed position. For some unknown reason, in about 10% of women it leans backwards instead, and adopts a retroverted and retroflexed position. This is not usually of significance but may sometimes cause dyspareunia if the ovaries are displaced too far and may predispose to infertility if the cervix points too much posteriorly.

In pregnancy the uterus undergoes further development as it comes to fulfil the purpose for which it was designed. The uterus of the nullipara is thus always smaller than that of the multiparous woman.

After the menopause in both nulliparous and multiparous women, the uterus atrophies and returns to its pre-adolescent size.

THE NON-PREGNANT UTERUS

Situation   The uterus lies in the true pelvis in an anteverted and anteflexed position. Its actual position is variable since it is dependent on how greatly the bladder, and to a lesser extent the rectum, is distended.

Shape   The shape resembles that of an English pear.

Size   7.5 cm long, 5 cm wide, 2.5 cm thick. The weight is approximately 57 g.

Gross structure (Fig. 8.1)

The cervix   forms the lower third of the uterus and has already been described in detail.

The isthmus   is the narrowed constriction about 7 mm thick lying between the body of the uterus and the cervix.

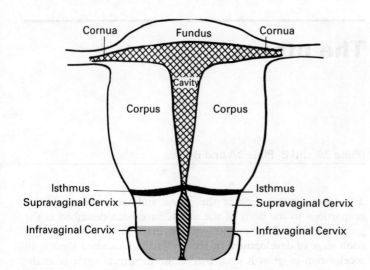

Fig. 8.1 Gross structure of the uterus.

The corpus or body	forms the upper two-thirds of the uterus and is that portion of the organ lying above the cervix.
The cornua	are the areas of the uterus where the fallopian tubes are inserted. The lumen of the tubes open into the uterine cavity.
The fundus	is the portion lying above and between the cornua.
The cavity	is the triangular-shaped potential hollow in the centre of the organ. The walls of the uterus normally lie in apposition.

Microscopic structure

Endometrium	A mucus membrane lining with secretory activity. Because it is influenced by the ovarian hormones, its appearance varies with each day of the menstrual cycle. During menstruation it is shed as far as the basal layer and is renewed on average every 28 days from the menarche to the menopause (see Ch. 9).
Myometrium	This is the muscle layer (Fig. 8.2) which makes up the chief bulk of the uterus during the period of active sexual life. Its structure differs before puberty and after the menopause. Involuntary muscle fibres are intermingled with areolar tissue, blood vessels lymphatic vessels and nerves.

Inner circular and outer longitudinal involuntary muscle fibres are continuous with those of the fallopian tubes and, together with involuntary circular muscle fibres forming the supporting ligaments

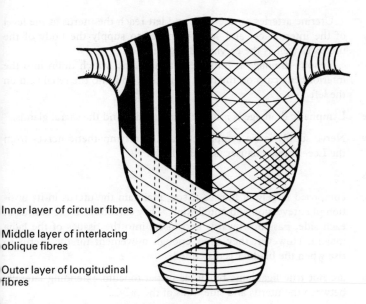

Inner layer of circular fibres

Middle layer of interlacing oblique fibres

Outer layer of longitudinal fibres

Fig. 8.2   Muscle structure of the uterus.

of the uterus, pass into the uterus to merge with the longitudinal and circular fibres there. These fibres all interlace to form spirals which pass in both clockwise and anticlockwise directions but form dense circles around the cornua and cervix. While it is impossible to define distinct muscle layers because the fibres are so intermingled, the middle strata, which contains the large blood vessels supplying the uterus, is much thicker than the layers on the inner and outer sides of it.

It seems that **uterine contractions** are partially initiated by the peristaltic waves in the fallopian tubes, and that the interlacing muscle fibres from the fallopian tubes and the ligaments, together with those of the uterus, become contractile as the result of oestrogen peaks during the menstrual cycle. Should there be any incoordination of muscle fibres from these three origins then dysmenorrhoea is a possible consequence. Conversely, when the muscle fibres act in co-ordination, the fimbriated end of the fallopian tube is brought into proximity with the ovary at the time of ovulation.

Perimetrium, or peritoneum covers the uterus quite smoothly and almost entirely. The areas which are excluded are: (1) those areas of cervix previously mentioned; and (2) a narrow strip of the lateral uterine walls. The peritoneum is attached quite firmly to the uterus except for an anterior portion of the isthmus, where its loose attachment allows the bladder to expand, and where it forms the uterovesical pouch. Posteriorly, peritoneum forms the pouch of Douglas.

Blood supply Ovarian arteries on the right and left from the abdominal aorta supply the fundus of the uterus. They pass downwards to meet the uterine artery of the corresponding side.

Uterine arteries on the right and left reach the uterus at the level of the internal os, and send branches to supply the body of the uterus as well as the cervix and vagina.

Venous drainage is into the ovarian veins, which drain into the inferior vena cava on the right hand side, and into the renal vein on the left.

Lymphatic drainage   Lymphatic drainage is into the internal iliac and the sacral glands.

Nerve supply   Nerve supply is via sympathetic and parasympathetic nerves from the Lee–Frankenhäuser (sacral) plexus.

Supports

The round ligaments,   composed largely of fibrous tissue, maintain the uterus in its position of anteversion and anteflexion. They extend from the cornua at each side, pass downwards and insert into the tissues of the labia majora. However, they allow enough movement for the uterus to rise when the bladder is distended.

The broad ligaments   are not true ligaments but folds of peritoneum extending laterally between the uterus and side walls of the pelvis.

The cardinal ligaments,
pubocervical ligaments and
uterosacral ligaments,   although described as supporting ligaments of the cervix, are obviously also uterine supports. Overstretching of these ligaments will result in prolapse of the uterus. They are composed of thickened bands of pelvic fascia, connective tissue and muscle fibres from the pelvic floor and uterus. In particular, the pubocervical ligaments are especially concerned with maintaining the angle between the cervix and the horizontal plane.

Functions
- To *prepare a bed for the fertilised ovum*
- To *nourish the fertilised ovum* for the gestation period
- To *expel the products of conception* at full term
- To *involute* following childbirth.

Relations   *Anterior:* as for the cervix. The intestines lie above the bladder and in front of the body of the uterus
Posterior: relations of the cervix and the uterosacral ligaments
Lateral: relations of the cervix, the fallopian tubes, ovaries and round ligaments
Superior: the intestines
Inferior: the vagina

The diagram showing relations of the vagina also shows relations of the cervix and the body of the uterus (Fig. 6.1).

THE PREGNANT UTERUS

Situation   By the 12th week of pregnancy, the uterus is rising out of the pelvis to become an abdominal organ. It is no longer anteverted and anteflexed but is becoming vertical. As it rises in the abdomen it leans towards the right. It reaches the umbilicus by the 24th week and the xiphisternum by the 36th week. Following the 36th week, the height of the fundus drops a little, because the fetal head starts to descend into the pelvis.

Shape   As the cavity of the uterus fills with the growing embryo, so the uterus becomes globular in shape. Between the 12th and 36th week, the isthmus trebles in length to accommodate it. The cavity becomes more ovoid as the fetus grows longer, and subsequently, as the fetal head descends into the pelvis, the uterus becomes more globular again.

Size   The number of weeks of gestation can be estimated by palpating the size of the uterus abdominally. At full term the uterus is 30 cm in length, 23 cm wide and 20 cm thick. Its weight has increased from 57 g to 1 kg. The hormone relaxin increases the ability of the uterus to distend but there is obviously much new growth as well.

Gross structure

The cervix   The changes of pregnancy have already been described.

The isthmus,   together with the cervix, develops to form the lower uterine segment.

Although there is strictly no anatomical distinction between the two poles, the upper and lower uterine segments will function quite differently during labour.

The cavity   is obviously no longer just potential space but is now filled with the products of conception.

Microscopic structure

Endometrium   Once the fertilised ovum has embedded, the uterine lining is renamed the **decidua** and becomes much thicker and more vascular than the non-pregnant endometrium. The glands become more vascular and their secretion is increased. These changes are affected by **oestrogen**, **progesterone** and **relaxin**.

Myometrium   Each muscle fibre increases ten times in length and at least three times in width. There is also a considerable amount of new muscle growth. Yet it should be recognised that the uterine muscle walls actually get thinner rather than thicker because of the gross enlargement of the organ. At the onset of labour the muscle wall is approximately 5–8 mm thick.

Rising oestrogen levels stimulate contractions of the myometrium and painless uterine contractions occur throughout pregnancy from the 8th week onwards. These are known as **Braxton Hicks** contractions and are preparing the uterine muscle for its action during labour. They are also believed to cause compression of the placenta and so propel a certain amount of blood to the fetus.

Relaxin inhibits contraction of the oestrogen-dominated myometrium and it is only when the oestrogen levels rise that the muscle becomes sensitive to oxytocin and labour contractions are initiated. The rising oestrogen levels are accompanied by reduced progesterone secretion.

Peritoneum grows at a corresponding rate with the uterus and continues to lie smoothly over it.

Blood supply and lymphatic drainage Both the blood and lymphatic vessels enlarge in order to keep pace with the growing uterus and its extra workload. In particular, the uterine arteries become less tortuous and the size of the lumen is increased. The ovarian veins become considerably enlarged in order to deal with the extra blood flow from the uterus.

Supports The greatest strain is put on the round ligaments. They can no longer maintain the uterus in its anteverted and anteflexed position and they thicken to such an extent during pregnancy that they can be palpated in the inguinal canal. It has been suggested that they hypertrophy in order to stabilise the uterus during labour, thus making uterine contractions more effective. Occasionally they become 'strained' and give rise to pain which can be confused with that caused by urinary tract infection, appendicitis or even concealed accidental antepartum haemorrhage. The collagenous and involuntary muscle content of the uterine ligaments is softened by the hormone relaxin and they all relax to some extent.

THE UTERUS IN LABOUR

The reasons as to why and when the uterus commences to contract and expel its contents have been a source of enquiry throughout the ages. Only one thing is certain, there is no single factor which initiates labour but several interdependent ones.

Causes of the onset of labour

Pressure on the cervix A well-fitting presenting part stimulates nerve endings in the cervix. Because the pressure of the presenting part causes the softened

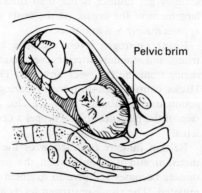

Pelvic brim

Fig. 8.3 Birth canal during first stage.

cervix to dilate at the internal os, the opposing actions of the upper and lower uterine segments now come into play. Because the cervix is dilating and shortening, the upper uterine segment begins to contract and retract.

Overdistention of the uterus Multiple pregnancy and hydramnios, conditions where the uterus is overdistended, both tend to be associated with the premature onset of labour. This suggests that nerve receptors in the uterine muscle are stimulated once the uterine contents are large enough. It does not, of course, account for the onset of *all* labours.

Progressive Braxton Hicks contractions Contractions commence in the cornua and are partially initiated by peristaltic action of the fallopian tubes. These painless but palpable contractions can be stimulated towards the end of pregnancy by abdominal examination and can be exacerbated if the midwife's hands are cold! Labour contractions are believed to be progressively strong Braxton Hicks contractions. It is also recognised that the administration of oxytocin in association with surgical rupture of the membranes will initiate labour contractions.

Hormonal factors Towards the end of pregnancy the fetal adrenal glands secrete rising levels of cortisol and androgenic hormones and these hormones stimulate the placenta to increase its oestrogenic and relaxin secretions. The production of progesterone does not change but the altered oestrogen/progesterone and relaxin balance reduces the relaxing effect of the uterine muscle. In turn this results in the release of prostaglandins which increase the ability of the uterine muscle to contract. This release of prostaglandins is associated with the release of oxytocin from the posterior pituitary gland. The dilatation of the lower uterine segment at the end of pregnancy is also believed to stimulate the release of oxytocin. The function of oxytocin, of course, is to stimulate uterine contractions.

Other factors Conditions such as fear and shock, febrile illnesses and eclampsia are all associated with the onset of labour, suggesting that physical and mental factors also play some part which we do not fully understand.

THE FIRST STAGE OF LABOUR

Definition The first stage of labour commences with uterine contractions which effect dilatation of the external os. It is completed when the cervix has opened widely enough to allow the fetal head to be delivered.

Effacement of the cervix 'Taking up' of the cervix has been described in Chapter 7. Suffice it to say here that in the primigravida this normally occurs during the last 2 weeks of pregnancy before the onset of labour. It does not occur in the multigravida until the fetal head begins to descend. Refer back to Figure 7.2 to see the demonstration of the dilatation of the cervix.

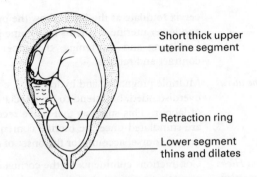

Short thick upper
uterine segment

Retraction ring

Lower segment
thins and dilates

Fig. 8.4 The uterus in labour:
first stage.

The 'show' As the internal os begins to dilate, so the placental membranes must inevitably become detached. As the chorion separates from the decidua small haemorrhages occur from the ruptured capillaries. Because the cervical canal dilates and becomes shorter, the operculum is discharged and both contribute to the vaginal discharge defined as the 'show'. The show is suggestive, but not indicative, that the first stage of labour has commenced.

Contraction and retraction of the upper uterine segment 1. *Contraction* implies a temporary shortening and thickening of muscle fibres during their active phase, then a return to original size and shape on cessation of activity, e.g. bulging of biceps muscles when lifting a heavy weight.

2. *Retraction* indicates a permanent partial shortening of muscle fibres which have been in a state of contraction. A certain amount of relaxation occurs, but the fibres do not return to their original length. Because they are shorter than they were originally, they are also thicker.

In labour, the muscles of the upper uterine segment contract and retract regularly, rhythmically and with increasing frequency, strength and duration. Contractions commence in the area of the cornua where they are strongest and then decrease in intensity as they pass to the lower uterine segment. With each contraction, muscle tone hardens the uterine walls in the upper segment, increases their thickness and diminishes the size of the cavity. The uterus changes its shape and position with each contraction. It becomes erect and pushes the abdominal wall forwards, bringing the axis of the uterus to lie at right angles to the plane of the pelvic brim. As a result of all these factors, the fetus is driven downwards and through the curve of the birth canal.

Dilatation and thinning of the lower uterine segment This thickening and shortening of the upper uterine segment, which drives the fetus downwards, achieves dilatation and thinning of the passive lower segment. As the contents of the uterine cavity are driven gradually into it, it relaxes and opens and the cervix is taken up to become one with it (see Figs 8.4 and 8.5A).

Retraction ring With progressive uterine contractions, the upper uterine segment becomes shorter and thicker and the lower uterine segment be comes thinner as it dilates. **Polarity** is the term used to describe this opposing but harmonious performance of the upper and lower uterine segments. The junction of the two segments is known as the **retraction ring**, but the effect of these two different activities is **not normally visible** on inspection of the abdomen. It can easily be seen, however, when the uterus is exposed at caesarean section.

Bandl's ring

In labours where there is prolonged or excessive opposing muscle action between the upper and lower uterine segments, the retraction ring occurs at a higher level in the uterus and becomes so pronounced that it **becomes visible abdominally**. It can be seen and palpated between the symphysis pubis and the umbilicus and is a serious indication of obstructed labour and a portent of uterine rupture.

Rupture of membranes

With each uterine contraction amniotic fluid is forced towards the weakest spot in the uterine walls, namely the dilating internal os. The placental membranes have been stripped from the area of attachment, allowing fluid to collect in that area and cause them to bulge; this forms the sac of forewaters. Providing that the head is well applied to the cervix, the forewaters act as a wedge in the dilating cervix and help it to open more widely with each contraction. With increasing dilatation there is proportionate detachment of the membranes and diminishing support for the forewaters. This lack of support, as well as the effect of relaxin on the placental membranes, associated with the increasing force of the descending fetal head, causes the membranes eventually to rupture and the amniotic fluid escapes.

Ideally, this rupture of the membranes occurs with full dilatation of the cervix immediately prior to the expulsion of the infant. The birth canal is then provided with a sterile douche immediately prior to the birth of the infant.

Early rupture of membranes

If the fetal head does not fit well, or in abnormal presentations where there is not a well-fitting presenting part, the membranes commonly rupture early in labour. The cervix may have only just commenced dilatation but uterine contractions force the amniotic fluid down freely around the presenting part and to collect below it. This results in the formation of a more sausage-shaped sac of forewaters and the membranes rupture early because they cannot withstand the tension caused by the amount of fluid within them. The fetal skull is then no longer protected from the pressure of the cervix by the sac of forewaters and so receives the direct pressure of the dilating cervix around the presenting part.

Anterior lip of cervix

Where the presenting part is not well applied to the cervix, the cervix is not withdrawn equally all the way round the head and a small anterior lip may prolong the first stage of labour. This is a common occurrence in the occipitoposterior position of the fetal head where the head does not descend with increasing flexion. Towards the end of the first stage of labour, the woman instinctively bears down with contractions, but clinical signs of full dilatation are not obvious. The condition can be diagnosed only by vaginal examination and when confirmed it is helpful to: 1) raise the foot of the bed so that pressure of the fetal head on the cervix is relieved, or it may be helpful to position the mother on her side – or even on all fours with her abdomen supported; 2) administer inhalational analgesia at the time of uterine contractions, or i.m.i. pethidine 100 mg if the cervix is oedematous and the woman distressed.

Cause of pain   There appears to be little relationship between the strength of uterine contractions and any pain which is sustained. For example, the tone of contractions in the third stage can be of equal intensity to some contractions in the first and second stage.

Pain is believed to be due to:

- *Ischaemia* of uterine muscle
- *Displacement* of other pelvic organs and tissues
- *Backache* which is largely the result of cervical dilatation when sensory fibres of sympathetic nerves from the sacral plexus are stimulated.

The management of the first stage of labour, the mother's position, occupation, who she wants with her, relief of pain etc. will all have been discussed with the midwife during the antenatal period.

SECOND STAGE

Definition   The second stage of labour commences with full dilatation of the cervix and is completed when the infant has been totally expelled from the uterus.

In this stage the **contractions become very characteristic in their expulsive nature** as well as being very strong (amplitude 60–80 mmHg). They continue to occur, as in the transitional stage, at about 2–3 minute intervals and last for about 1 minute. The **fetus is now driven downwards by the grossly retracted upper uterine segment**, through the widely opened cervix and birth canal. He is driven by **fetal axis pressure** downwards and backwards, perpendicular to the pelvic brim.

Posteriorly

The ischiorectal fat and the pelvic floor muscles are pushed downwards in front of the presenting part so that the perineum bulges, stretches and thins, the rectum is compressed and the anus becomes widely dilated. It is very important now that the woman has been taught to relax these muscles since, if they remain tense

- *Labour will be prolonged* because the fetus cannot advance
- *The tissues are more likely to be damaged* by pressure of the head
- *Episiotomy may be necessary* or spontaneous laceration occur.

Anteriorly

The pelvic floor muscles are drawn upwards over the descending fetal head, together with the empty bladder because of its attachment to the lower uterine segment by peritoneum. If the bladder is full it will: (1) cause obstruction to the fetal head; (2) inhibit uterine contractions; and (3) be compressed, with consequent trauma. It should therefore be emptied by catheterisation between uterine contractions but, as the urethra is elongated and the lumen narrowed and the fetal head is causing compression, the procedure is a difficult one.

Between uterine contractions the fetal head recedes and then advances a little further with each contraction until it is crowned, i.e. the widest transverse diameter of the fetal skull has distended the perineum. Once the head has been delivered there is a short rest and then a further uterine contraction expedites delivery of the anterior and then the posterior shoulder.

With the delivery of the infant's body there is further contraction and retraction of the upper uterine segment and the slow delivery of the body aids the separation of the placenta.

THIRD STAGE

Placental separation

The placenta does not normally start to separate with uterine contractions during the first and early second stages of labour because the placental site must be reduced to approximately half its original size before any separation is possible. Obviously, while the fetus is still in the uterus there can be no reduction in the size of the uterus. As the infant's body is being expelled in the second stage of labour there is a marked reduction in the length of the uterus, the thickness of its muscle walls increases and the size of its cavity is reduced. Separation of the placenta normally begins when the placental site is reduced to about half its size. It usually commences in the centre and extends to its circumference. Not being made of elastic tissue, the placenta is peeled off the uterine wall.

To bring about this separation another important factor is also

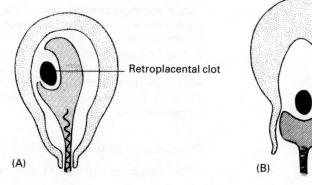

Retroplacental clot

(A) (B)

Fig. 8.5 The uterus in labour: (A) second stage: separation and descent of placenta (B) third stage: expulsion of placenta. Uterus further contracts and retracts to control haemorrhage.

involved. When the placental site is reduced in size, the placenta itself becomes compressed so that blood in the intervillous spaces is forced back into the maternal veins of the decidua. These over-distended veins are then compressed between the retracted uterine muscle fibres on one side and the placenta on the other. With the next uterine contraction these congested blood vessels rupture and bleed into the decidua, causing a blood clot and also tearing the layer of perforated cells between the decidua and the myometrium (the **layer of Nitabuch**). The placenta thus separates, leaving only the basal layer of endometrial cells to promote regeneration of the endometrium.

A really effective uterine contraction will not only cause placental separation, but will also expel it into the lower uterine segment and upper vagina almost immediately after the birth of the infant. More commonly, there is a short period of relaxation of uterine muscle, during which time there may be a little blood loss from the intervillous spaces and from the maternal blood vessels.

Placental expulsion

When the placenta has separated, it folds slightly but remains in the uterine cavity because the membranes are still attached to the decidua. With the next uterine contraction the placenta is pushed down to the lower uterine segment and the membranes are peeled away by its weight as it descends. Because the lower uterine segment is now dilated with the placenta, the upper segment contracts and retracts to become even shorter and thicker. In this way, the muscle fibres continue to exert pressure on the uterine blood vessels and haemorrhage from the placental site is controlled.

It is possible to appreciate the high tone of the muscular contraction and retraction simply by placing a flat hand on the abdomen. The uterus can be felt to rise and become a firm hard mass with the consistency of a cricket ball.

At the end of the third stage of labour the uterus measures approximately 15 cm in length 10 cm in width and 7.5 cm in depth.

Methods of placental separation

Placental separation may occur in one of two ways:

Schultze method

This is the most usual method of placental separation and is the mechanism which has just been described. Because the centre of the placenta separates first, it folds in the centre as it descends and moves, fetal surface first, through the birth canal to the vulva. On examination a small clot, the retroplacental clot, is found on the maternal surface in the central area where separation first occurred. There is minimal postpartum blood loss when the placenta separates this way.

Matthews Duncan method

When the placenta is situated with its lower border encroaching into the lower uterine segment, increasing separation of the lower border is inevitable as the lower segment distends during the first and second stages of labour. In the third stage of labour, when separation is complete, the placenta descends by slipping sideways, lower border first. It is the maternal surface which therefore presents first at the vulva. Expulsion is associated with a little heavier blood loss than with the Schultze method and there is no retroplacental blood clot.

Placenta accreta In very rare instances, placental separation is impossible because of an abnormality in the spongy layer of the decidua, where there is no layer of Nitabuch. The chorionic villi therefore embed not only into the endometrium but also into the muscle of the uterine wall. Attempts at manual removal of the placenta are impossible and the placenta is either left in situ to calcify or, following consultation with the woman and her husband, hysterectomy may be performed.

Control of haemorrhage
(Fig. 8.6)

Compression When the mechanism of placental separation is completed, the placenta is pushed into the lower uterine segment by further contractions in the upper segment. The lower segment being dilated results in the upper segment contracting and retracting still further to become even shorter and thicker (polarity of the uterus). In this way, the muscle fibres apply pressure to the blood vessels and haemorrhage from the placental site is controlled.

Because of the gross contraction and retraction of the upper uterine segment, the cavity of the uterus is now closed with the walls lying in apposition. This exerts further pressure on the placental site and assists the compression of blood sinuses there (Fig. 8.6).

Coagulation During and immediately following the third stage of labour there is an increased tendency for blood in the large uterine vessels to clot and this aids control of haemorrhage at the placental site.

Oxytocic drugs An i.m.i. of Syntometrine 1 ml is the most usual drug given currently to prevent and/or control postpartum haemorrhage. Syntometrine consists of 0.5 mg of ergometrine combined with 5 units of synthetic oxytocin. It should be remembered that while synthetic oxytocin acts within 2 minutes, the action of ergometrine is delayed for at least 5 minutes. The placenta therefore needs to be delivered

Fig. 8.6 Control of haemorrhage by uterine muscle. Contracted fibres cause compression of blood vessels: (A) relaxed uterine muscle fibres surrounding blood vessel (B) contracted fibres show 'living ligature' action.

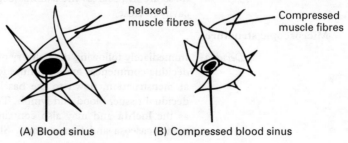

Relaxed muscle fibres

Compressed muscle fibres

(A) Blood sinus   (B) Compressed blood sinus

within 5 minutes of its administration, for after that time the cervix will close. The decision as to whether the drug is to be given with the crowning of the head or the birth of the anterior shoulder, or even given at all, is dependent upon the way in which the mother and the midwife decide to manage the third stage of labour.

THE UTERUS IN THE PUERPERIUM

The puerperium is a period of from 6–8 weeks following childbirth, during which time the genital organs return to their pre-pregnant state, lactation should be established and the new infant should be accepted into the family. The uterus, which developed over a 40-week period during pregnancy, has now a much shorter time in which to make regressive changes. These changes are described as **involution**.

Situation   Immediately following the third stage of labour the fundus of the uterus is found about halfway between the symphysis pubis and the umbilicus. Within the next 24 hours the lower uterine segment regains its tone, and consequently pushes up the fundus to the level of the umbilicus. If the uterus is then palpated on each successive day, it is found to be a fingerbreadth lower in the abdomen at each examination. By the 10th day of the puerperium it can no longer be palpated abdominally, because anteversion and anteflexion are almost complete. Before the uterus is palpated the mother should be asked to empty her bladder. However, this examination is rarely carried out as a daily general policy in the UK today.

Shape   When the placenta has been expelled the uterus contracts and retracts and becomes globular in shape. As involution takes place the cavity becomes smaller, and 6 weeks following delivery the uterus has returned to its original, pear-like shape.

Size   At the end of labour, the uterus is approximately 15 cm long, 10 cm wide, 7.5 cm thick and weighs 0.9 kg. During the first week of the puerperium it loses 0.45 kg in weight and a further 0.2 kg in the second week. At the end of the puerperium it is once again 7.5 cm long, 5 cm wide, 2.5 cm thick and weighs 57 g.

Gross structure   The changes in the cervix have already been described and while these are in progress the isthmus begins to reform and the uterine cavity to close.

Microscopic structure

Decidua   Immediately following the delivery of the placenta, the shedding of decidua commences and continues for about 10 days. It is shed, as at menstruation, down to the basal layer and consists largely of decidual tissue, blood and lymph. This vaginal discharge is known as the **lochia** and may also contain, at first, meconium, lanugo, vernix caseosa and liquor amnii. Shreds of chorion may also be expelled if not delivered with the placenta. As the uterus contracts in order to expel blood clots, 'after-pains' are often experienced. These pains can be relieved by mild analgesic drugs, and 0.5 mg ergometrine given orally or by intramuscular injection will produce stronger uterine contractions to expel the clots.

Regeneration of the endometrium is slow to commence and it is almost 2 weeks before regrowth of the epithelial tissue occurs. The process is not complete until 6 weeks after delivery. The placental site takes about 8 weeks to heal. In comparison with regeneration of the basal endometrium following menstruation this is a relatively long process, but the levels of oestrogen during these weeks are proportionally low.

In theory, urinalysis could be carried out to estimate the rate of involution, the amount of urea in the urine being the result of tissue breakdown.

There is no change in the endometrium of the isthmus and cervix as the tissues there did not proliferate and become secretory during pregnancy.

Myometrium
The **hypertrophy** (increased thickness) and **hyperplasia** (increased number) of muscle fibres which occurred during pregnancy now needs to be reduced. Following the third stage of labour, these muscles continue to contract and retract and produce **ischaemia** as the blood vessels with which they are interlaced are compressed. This reduced blood supply results in atrophy of fibrous and elastic tissue which is then broken down by **phagocytosis**. Some elastic tissue remains unaffected by the process and helps to account for the larger uterus associated with the multipara.

Proteolytic enzymes are also released to aid the process of muscle reduction. Lysin, a cell-dissolving substance contained in blood serum, breaks down muscle fibres and all these waste products of myometrium are circulated in the blood and excreted by the kidneys in the urine.

Peritoneum
At the end of the third stage, the peritoneum lies in a wrinkled manner over the uterus and its appendages but it shrinks at the same rate as the uterus and returns to become a smooth outer covering.

Blood supply
Because of the pressure exerted by the retracted uterine muscle fibres, the blood in the uterine vessels clots. Simultaneously with absorption of this clot, new smaller blood vessels develop within the old ones, resulting in their re-canalisation and a less abundant blood supply to the now non-pregnant uterus. The blood returns to its normal viscosity.

Supports
The supporting ligaments of the uterus, as well as the pelvic floor muscles, have all lost some tone during pregnancy and labour and the sooner ambulation and generalised activity can be recommenced the better. If any of these structures is permanently weakened, then stress incontinence, dyspareunia and prolapse of the uterus are possible sequelae to childbirth.

POSTNATAL EXAMINATION

This examination has been mentioned in previous chapters. It can be considered more fully here.

Appointment Before her discharge from the maternity unit, the mother should be given an appointment for the postnatal clinic if she is to return to hospital for the examination. More often, specialist follow-up is not necessary and her general practitioner will be asked to see her. In this instance, the mother should be advised to make an appointment to see him when her baby is 6 weeks old. She should also be advised to see him before this time if she feels concerned about herself or the baby.

Objective
- To assess the woman's general state of physical and mental health
- To detect any condition arising from her pregnancy or labour which affects her well-being.

General examination

Enquire as to her general well-being, the well-being of the baby and how they are settling together as a family

Assess her (1) weight, (2) haemoglobin, (3) blood pressure and (4) carry out urinalysis

Examination 1. *Examine the breasts*. Enquire about adequacy of lactation and if baby is feeding satisfactorily. Ensure that there are no signs of breast infection and that there are no 'lumps'. If lactation has been suppressed it is equally important that the breasts are examined. Remind the mother to carry out regular self-examination of her breasts.

2. *Palpate the abdomen* to elicit that the uterus is no longer palpable. Assess the muscle tone of the abdominal wall.

3. *Examine the legs* for signs of varicosities and oedema. Advise as necessary or refer to the appropriate clinic.

Ask specific questions, relating to:

- Vaginal discharge
- Resumption of menstruation
- Increased frequency of micturition
- Dysuria
- Stress urgency or stress incontinence
- Backache
- Pelvic discomfort
- Resumption of sexual intercourse, excluding any difficulties such as vaginismus, frigidity or dyspareunia.

Vaginal examination This is to assess:

- Condition of the vulva
- Healing of the perineal and vaginal lacerations
- Condition of the cervix, that it is healthy and that there is no cervical erosion. A cervical smear test may be carried out

- Whether the uterus is anteverted and anteflexed and has returned to its normal size
- The tone of the pelvic floor muscles. Exclude conditions such as cystocele, urethrocele, rectocele and any degree of uterine prolapse. Note any stress incontinence.

During the examinations, natural conversation will also provide an opportunity to assess the mother's mental and emotional state. Following full examination, any advice regarding referral to other hospital clinics, possible counselling or treatment can be discussed.

Contraception Before leaving the clinic the mother should be reminded that, unless she is *fully* breast feeding (i.e. 3–4-hourly by day and also at night) or wishes to become pregnant quite quickly, it is advisable to commence the use of contraceptives if she has not already done so (see Ch. 11). Referral can be made to a family planning clinic if she wishes.

REVISION QUESTIONS

Describe the shape, size and structure of the uterus at term. What changes does it undergo during each stage of labour?

Describe the structure of the uterus, the changes which take place in it during pregnancy and the way in which the uterus prevents haemorrhage after the birth of the baby.

Describe the supports of the uterus. How may they be damaged in labour? How can the risk of such damage be reduced?

Describe the uterine muscle and its action in all the stages of labour.

Describe the anatomy of the body of the uterus. Describe the muscle action of the uterus in the third stage of labour.

What changes take place in the uterus during the puerperium? What may interfere with normal involution?

Outline the anatomy of the body of the uterus. Describe the behaviour of its musculature in the three stages of labour.

Define:

1st stage of labour
2nd stage of labour
3rd stage of labour.

About how long does each stage normally last?

What part is played by hormones in the stimulation of uterine contractions?

REFERENCES AND FURTHER READING

Books and reports
Flint C 1982 Sensitive midwifery. Heinemann, London
Garcia J et al 1985 Midwives confined. Labour ward policies and routine procedures. Mios conference report

Inch S 1983 Birthrights. Hutchinson, London

Macfarlane A 1977 The psychology of childbirth. Fontana, London

O'Driscoll K, Meagner D 1986 Active management of labour: the Dublin experience, 2nd edn. Baillière Tindall, London

Prince J, Adams M E 1987 The psychology of childbirth, 2nd edn. Churchill Livingstone, Edinburgh

Articles

Biancuzzo M 1991 The patient observer: does the hands and knees position during labour help to rotate the OPP of the fetus? Birth 18(1): 40–43

Bonnar J, McNicol G P, Douglas A S 1970 Coagulation and fibrinolytic mechanisms during and after normal childbirth. British Medical Journal ii: 200–203

Brandt M 1933 The mechanism and management of the third stage of labour. American Journal of Obstetrics and Gynecology 25: 662–667

Dunn P M 1991 Francis Mauriceau (1637–1709) and maternal posture for parturition. Archives of Diseases of Childbirth 66(1): 78–79

Editorial 1990 Stand and deliver. Lancet i: 761–762

Edwards ? 1990 National Childbirth Trust Study Day on the 3rd Stage. AIMS Quarterly Journal 1(4): 7

Garcia J, Garforth S 1989 Labour and delivery routines in English consultant maternity units. Midwifery 5(4): 155–162

Gardosi J 1989 Alternative positions in the second stage of labour. British Journal of Obstetrics and Gynaecology 6(11): 1290–1296

Gardosi J, Hutson N, B-Lynch C 1989 Randomised controlled trial of squatting in the second stage of labour (and letters in reply) Lancet ii: 74–77; 700

Levy V 1981 The midwife's management of the third stage of labour. Nursing Mirror Occasional Papers no 5

Marttila M, Kajanoja P, Ylikorkala O 1983 Maternal half-sitting position in the second stage of labour. Journal of Perinatal Medicine 11(6): 286–289

Metcalfe E, Rathbone A 1988 The postnatal examination. Update (March 1): 1868–1875

McFadyen I R 1969 Uterovaginal prolapse 1. Nursing Times 65: 167–169

Narroll F 1961 Positions of women in childbirth. American Journal of Obstetrics and Gynecology 82: 943

Odent MR 1990 Position in delivery: the need to be upright. Lancet 335: 1166

Prendiville W J, Harding J E, Elbourne D R, Stirrat G M 1988 The Bristol third stage trial: active versus physiological management of third stage of labour. British Medical Journal 297: 1295–1300

Roberts J et al 1983 The effects of maternal position in uterine contractility and efficiency. Birth 10: 243

Russell J G 1982 The rationale of primitive delivery positions. British Journal of Obstetrics and Gynaecology 89: 712–715

Sadler S 1985 Third stage management. New Generation 4(2): 22

Stewart P, Spiby H 1988 Posture in labour. British Journal of Obstetrics and Gynaecology 96(1): 1258–1260

Stewart P, Spiby H 1989 Randomised study of sitting position for delivery using a newly designed obstetric chair. British Journal of Obstetrics and Gynaecology 96(3): 327–333

Waldenström U, Gottvall K 1991 A randomised trial of birthing stool or conventional semi-recumbent position. Birth 18(1): 5–10

9 The fallopian tubes and ovaries

(Plate 2A and B, Plate 3A, Plate 6)

THE FALLOPIAN TUBES

Situation   Each tube extends from the cornua of the uterus, travels towards the side walls of the pelvis, then turns downwards and backwards before reaching it. The tubes lie within the broad ligament.

Shape   They are tubular, as their name implies. The lumen of each tube communicates with the cavity of the uterus at its proximal end and the peritoneal cavity at its distal end. There is therefore a direct communication between the vaginal orifice in the vulva and the peritoneal cavity, which increases the risk of ascending genital tract infection.

Size   The length of each tube is approximately 10 cm.
The diameter varies in each part of the tube:

- *Interstitial portion* 1 mm
- *Isthmus* 2.5 mm
- *Ampulla and infundibulum* each 6 mm.

Gross structure (Fig. 9.1)

The interstitial portion   lies within the wall of the uterus and is 2.5 cm in length.

The isthmus   is also 2.5 cm in length. It is the narrowest portion of the tube and acts as a reservoir for spermatozoa because the temperature is lower there than in the rest of the tube. The lumen of the isthmus is under hormonal control and is contracted or dilated according to stimulating hormones which also affect the condition of the uterine endometrium.

The ampulla   is the widened out area of the tube where fertilisation normally occurs. It is 5 cm in length.

The infundibulum or fimbriated end   is the terminal and distal portion of the tube which turns backwards and downwards and ends in finger-like projections (**fimbriae**) which surround the orifice of the tube. One fimbria lies in closer proximity to the ovary than the others.

Microscopic structure

Ciliated epithelium   forms the lining of the tube. As the result of ovarian hormone

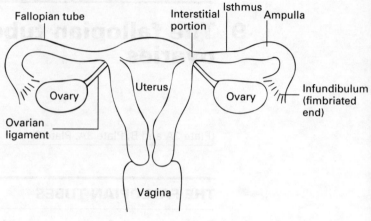

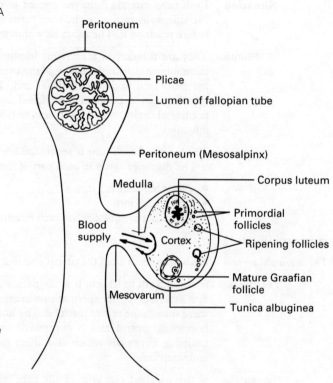

Fig. 9.1 The fallopian tube and ovary: (A) gross structure (B) relationship of fallopian tube and ovary and structure of the ovary.

stimulation it undergoes very slight hypertrophy during the menstrual cycle and its secretions and deposits of glycogen are increased just prior to menstruation. It undergoes decidual changes if the fertilised ovum embeds in the tube.

The epithelium is arranged in folds, **plicae**, which slow down the passage of the fertilised ovum, allowing it to develop in preparation for its embedding in the uterus. There is a more pronounced arrangement of plicae in the ampulla.

Connective tissue   lies beneath the epithelium.

Muscle is arranged in two layers:

1. An **inner layer** of involuntary circular muscle fibres
2. An **outer layer** of involuntary longitudinal fibres which continue into the body of the uterus. It is largely their peristaltic action which propels the ovum towards the uterus. Contractions of the longitudinal fibres bring the fimbria nearer to the ovary at the time of ovulation. Uterine contractions are a continuation of this tubal peristaltic action.

Peritoneum   hangs over the tubes but is absent on their inferior surface.

Blood supply   The blood supply comes from the uterine and ovarian arteries; venous return is by corresponding veins.

The infundibulum has a particularly rich supply and blood vessels there are intermingled with muscle fibres. At the time of ovulation, the blood vessels become engorged and give the fimbriae increased power of movement so that they can range over the ovary and waft the ovum into the lumen.

Lymphatic drainage   The lymphatic drainage is into the lumbar glands.

Nerve supply   The nerve supply is from the ovarian plexus.

Supports   This is provided by the **infundibulopelvic ligaments**. These are formed from folds of the broad ligament and run from the infundibulum of the tube to the side walls of the pelvis.

Function   The tube forms a canal through which the ovum and sperm can pass and unite and where the fertilised ovum can commence early development.

Relations   *Anterior*: ⎫
Posterior: ⎬   the peritoneal cavity and the intestines
Superior: ⎭
Inferior: the broad ligament and the ovaries
Lateral: infundibulopelvic ligaments and round ligaments
Medial: the uterus

Ectopic gestation

An ectopic gestation is a pregnancy which develops outside the uterus. This most commonly occurs in the fallopian tube. The causes of a tubal pregnancy have not really been determined, but an obstructed tube is obviously a predisposing factor. There is also said to be a higher incidence in those women who use an intrauterine contraceptive device.

If the embryo develops in the isthmus, the narrowest part of the tube, it soon erodes through the thin layer of tissues in the embedding process, ruptures the tube and opens up large blood vessels, causing an intraperitoneal haemorrhage. The condition is then known as a **ruptured ectopic gestation** and constitutes an acute abdominal catastrophe. Blood transfusion followed by prompt surgical operation, in which the tube is excised, become essentially life-saving operations.

THE OVARIES

Development

The ovaries originate from the same embryonic structure as the suprarenal glands and the male testes, but they still lie above the pelvic brim at the time of birth and do not descend until the cavity of the pelvis deepens during childhood. There is very little development of the infantile ovary until the onset of the menarche and its appearance and structure then differ according to a woman's age and the phase of her menstrual cycle.

Situation (frontispiece)

The two ovaries lie within the peritoneal cavity in a small depression of the posterior wall of the broad ligament. They are situated at the fimbriated end of the fallopian tube, at about the level of the pelvic brim.

Shape

The ovaries are small, almond-like organs, dull white in colour and with a corrugated surface.

Size

3 cm × 2 cm × 1 cm. Weight 5–8 g.

Gross structure
(see Fig. 9.1B)

This varies with the age of the woman.

Birth to puberty

The organs are smooth, dull white and rather solid in consistency.

Menstrual phase

Between puberty and the menopause the organs are larger and are rather irregular on the surface, more like a walnut than an almond.

Post-menopausal phase

The ovaries become smaller and shrunken and are covered with scar tissue where, month after month, the graafian follicles have ruptured.

Microscopic structure
(Fig. 9.1B)

Germinal epithelium

is another name for the peritoneum which encloses the ovary.

Tunica albuginea

is the tough, fibrous outer coat.

Cortex

consists mostly of vascular fibrous tissue stroma in which **graafian follicles** are embedded. These follicles each contain an **ovum** and can be found at varying degrees of development. The **corpus luteum** is the scar tissue which forms after a follicle has burst. The cortex is, therefore, the 'working part' of the ovary.

Medulla

is the central portion and point of entry for blood vessels, lymphatics and nerves. It consists chiefly of fibrous and elastic tissue.

Life cycle of a primordial follicle

Primordial follicle — At birth, the cortex of the ovary contains about 200 000 primordial follicles, each of which contains a primordial sex cell. Some follicles may attempt to mature before puberty but they are normally unsuccessful and degenerate.

Graafian follicle (Fig. 9.2) — With the onset of puberty several follicles attempt to mature simultaneously during the first half of the menstrual cycle. One is more successful than the others, fills with fluid, reaches a diameter of least 10 mm and then rises to the surface of the ovary. During this process, the first meiotic division takes place in the nucleus of the primordial sex cell. The graafian follicle ruptures through the surface of the ovary and releases the follicular fluid and the ovum.

Corpus luteum — is the shell left by the ruptured graafian follicle. It fills with blood clots and then fibrosis commences. After 10 days it ceases to increase in size and begins to form scar tissue.

Corpus albicans — is the name given to the structure as it continues to fibrose.

Corpus fibrosum — is the structure in its final stage of fibrosis. It is the increasing number of scars left by the occurrence of each ovulation that gives the surface of the ovary its post-menopausal scarred appearance.

Blood supply — The blood is supplied from the ovarian arteries; venous drainage is into the ovarian veins.

Lymphatic drainage — Lymphatic drainage is into the lumbar glands.

Nerve supply — The nerve supply is from the ovarian plexus.

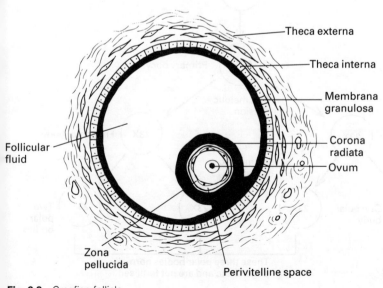

Fig. 9.2 Graafian follicle.

Supports   The fossa in which the ovary lies. Where it is attached to the broad ligament is called the **mesovarium**. The broad ligament which extends between the fallopian tubes and the ovary is known as the **mesosalpinx**.

Function   To produce ova for fertilisation, oestrogen and progesterone.

Relations (Fig. 9.1B)   *Anterior*: the broad ligament
Lateral: the fallopian tube

THE PRODUCTION OF MATURE OVA
(OOGENESIS) (Fig. 9.3)

Primordial sex cells   These are first seen in the embryonic ectoderm of the yolk sac and migrate to the germinal epithelium of the ovary at about the 6th week of intrauterine life. Each female primordial sex cell, (oogonium), is surrounded by pre-granulosa cells which protect and nourish it and, together, the cells form a primordial follicle.

Primordial follicles   These migrate to the stroma of the ovarian cortex where they make up the 200 000 or so which are present there at birth. Some attempt further development during intrauterine life and during childhood but normally none reach maturity. Only about 40 000 remain when the girl reaches puberty. At puberty one follicle completes the

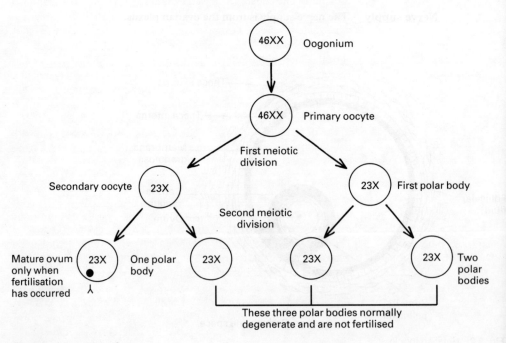

Fig. 9.3   Maturation of ovum.

maturation process during each menstrual cycle and is known as a **graafian follicle**. The sex cell which it contains is a **primary oocyte**.

Primary oocyte

The nucleus of the primary oocyte contains 23 pairs of chromosomes (**diploid chromosomes**). One pair of chromosomes are the **sex-determining chromosomes** and are designated XX. The other chromosomes are known as **autosomes**.

Each chromosome is composed of two **chromatids**.

Each pair of chromosomes therefore has four chromatids.

Chromatids carry the **genes**, genetic material commonly called **DNA** (**deoxyribonucleic acid**) and protein materials.

Genetic material conveys inherited appearance and characteristics from parents to their children.

First meiotic division

Mitosis occurs in the ovary while the graafian follicle is maturing. It is completed before ovulation occurs.

The nucleus of the oocyte or **ovum** divides in such a way that the pairs of chromosomes are split and two cells each containing 23 chromosomes are produced by the division. One cell retains most of the cytoplasm and is therefore larger than the other. This cell is the **secondary oocyte**.

The smaller cell is known as the **first polar body** and is extruded into the **perivitelline space** of the graafian follicle. This first polar body sometimes reproduces itself. They will normally both degenerate.

In this first meiotic division, which brings about the **haploid** number of chromosomes in the secondary oocyte and the first polar body, there is also an interchange of the chromatids and their genetic material. Each chromosome retains one chromatid but interchanges the other. The two cells therefore have the same number of chromosomes but a different pattern of genetic material. This interchange is essential if family likenesses and inherited characteristics are to be reproduced without identical likenesses occurring.

A similar reduction in the chromosomes of the spermatozoa is brought about during their maturation process so that at fertilisation the 23 chromosomes of the secondary oocyte are united with the 23 chromosomes of the sperm and the human cell pattern of 46 chromosomes is restored.

Secondary oocyte

A second meiotic division is usually brought about only when the head of the sperm penetrates the zona pellucida which surrounds the oocyte (ovum). The secondary oocyte divides to form the **mature ovum** and another polar body.

Two or three polar bodies and one mature ovum, all containing different genetic material, have now been formed (Fig. 9.3). **The three polar bodies normally degenerate**.

The mature fertilised ovum commences embryonic development. The production of spermatozoa will be covered in the next chapter, but it should be noted here that, in the female, the sex chromosomes XX are homozygous, while the male carries heterozygous, sex-determining chromosomes. The 'X' of his pair is a female-determining cell while the 'Y', the smaller of the pair, is a male-determining cell.

It is also of interest to note that, while the mature spermatozoon is the smallest cell in the body, varying between 52 μm and 62 μm in length, the ovum is the largest. When the ovum is mature it can reach 142 μm in diameter. (1 μm = 0.001 mm).

THE MENSTRUAL CYCLE (Plate 6, Fig. 9.4.)

This is a cycle of events occurring in the ovary which produces changes not only in the uterus but in the female body as a whole. Its objective is to release an ovum in preparation for fertilisation at approximately 4-week intervals and to prepare the uterus and the whole female body for its reception and development.

The cycle is dominated by the anterior pituitary gland but the factors which cause it to stimulate the gonads at the time of puberty are not fully understood.

It is recognised that:

1. There is some **neurohormonal control** of the anterior pituitary gland by the **hypothalamus** and the cycle can be influenced by emotional factors such as a change of job, move to a different country, death of a loved one, etc.

2. While the **anterior pituitary gland** regulates the secretions

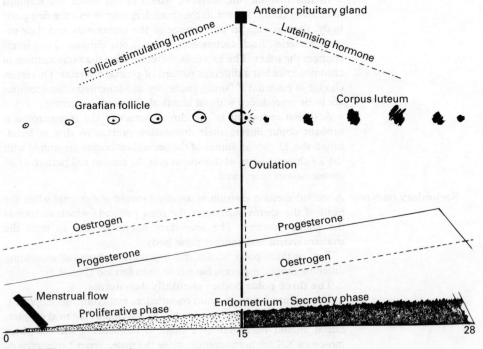

Fig. 9.4 The menstrual cycle.

by the ovary of oestrogen and progesterone, it is itself regulated by these secretions. There appears to be a fine balance and inter-dependence between them.

The length of the 'average' menstrual cycle is 28 days and this is divided into four phases.

Oestrogens   The secretion of oestrogen is controlled by Follicle Stimulating Hormone (FSH) and Luteinising Hormone (LH) from the anterior pituitary gland. The anterior pituitary gland is under direct control of the hypothalamus and is therefore influenced by stimulus from the mind as well as the body.

The principal oestrogen produced is **oestradiol**, with **oestrone** and **oestriol** present in smaller quantities.

Oestrogens are produced by theca cells and granulosa cells of the graafian follicle and by the corpus luteum during the first 12 weeks of pregnancy, then by the placenta. Oestrone is also produced by the adrenal glands and is the main type of oestrogen found in post-menopausal women.

At puberty oestrogens produce development of the secondary sexual characteristics in the female, i.e. they:

- Increase the length of the long bones and close the epiphyses
- Develop the glandular tissue of the breast
- Increase deposits of the subcutaneous fat which gives the female figure its curves
- Bring the structures of the external genitalia to their female adult status.

After puberty they:

- Stimulate the growth of the endometrium and increase its vascularity
- Promote regeneration of the endometrium after menstruation
- Increase the cervical mucus and reduce its viscosity at the time of ovulation
- Cause proliferation of the vaginal epithelium and ensure that the cells are packed with glycogen.

Natural oestrogens from the ovary and the adrenals lower the levels of cholesterol and the incidence of coronary heart disease in women, whereas synthetic oestrogens increase the level of fibrin and therefore the clotting power of blood and cause a predisposition to thromboembolic diseases, as well as coronary heart disease. They also cause a rise in blood pressure.

Progesterone   Progesterone is produced largely in the second half of the menstrual cycle, when it is secreted by the corpus luteum. It is also produced in tiny quantities by the granulosa cells of the corpus luteum, which also produce small quantities of oestrogen. Its main functions are concerned with tissues which have already been receptive to oestogen.

In the second half of the menstrual cycle, the secretory phase:

1. The endometrial glands become tortuous and secrete more mucus and a fluid which is rich in glycogen
2. Water is retained in the endometrium and the stroma becomes waterlogged
3. Progesterone:
   - makes the cervical mucus much more tenacious before and after ovulation
   - acts on the muscle fibres of the fallopian tube, increasing muscle tone
   - reduces the frequency of peristaltic contractions, causing vaginal epithelium to desquamate, and depletes epithelial cells of glycogen
   - increases the vascularity of the breasts and causes proliferation of mammary tissue
   - increases water and sodium retention in body tissues.

Growth of the graafian follicle is stimulated by FSH and small amounts of LH (oestradiol).

Initially, rising oestradiol levels inhibit FSH. Then at mid-cycle there is a sudden secretory surge of FSH and LH.

Phases of the menstrual cycle

Regenerative phase

During the first few days of this phase, the endometrium of the uterus is shed right down to the basal layer and initially, the rising oestrogen level inhibits the follicle stimulating hormone.

The **anterior pituitary gland** then releases **follicle stimulating hormone**, causing several **graafian follicles** to fill with fluid and increase in size. This results in a rising level of **oestrogen** circulating in the bloodstream. The alteration in hormone balance causes new growth of endometrium of the uterus. In the normal event, all the follicles except one fail to mature and degenerate. The follicle which survives reaches a diameter of 1.5–2 cm and rises to the surface of the ovary. If the length of a woman's menstrual cycle is shorter or longer than 28 days it is this regenerative phase that is variable.

Ovulation

There comes a time when, as the result of its increasing size, the graafian follicle will rupture, although the rupture is more like a slow leaking of fluid rather than an instant deflation. Relaxin aids the rupture by softening the follicle membrane. With rising oestrogen levels, LH is released from the anterior pituitary gland, resulting in a surge at mid-cycle of both FSH and LH.

With the rupture of the follicle, the ovum is released (**ovulation**) and the oestrogen level decreases.

Secretory phase

The ruptured follicle, now known as the **corpus luteum**, is stimulated by LH from the anterior pituitary gland (FSH being simultaneously withdrawn). The corpus luteum now begins to increase in size and to produce progesterone in increasing amounts. This further change in hormone balance stimulates the uterus to prepare its lining for the reception of a fertilised ovum and it undergoes the following secretory changes:

- The endometrium becomes much thicker and more spongy
- The blood supply is increased
- There is increased activity of the secretory glands
- Mineral salts and glucose are deposited.

Menstruation   If the ovum is not fertilised, it dies within 12–24 hours and the anterior pituitary gland withdraws luteinising hormone after 14–15 days. Preparations for pregnancy cease and the endometrium is shed with the menstrual flow. Some hours before the onset of menstrual bleeding, the blood vessels become constricted by the congested endometrial tissues. Blood is extruded from the capillary vessels causing necrosis and then shedding of the endometrium. As LH is withdrawn, the anterior pituitary gland once again prepares for pregnancy by releasing FSH, and another regenerative phase begins. Day 1 of the menstrual cycle is the first day of endometrial bleeding.

Hormonal activity during the menstrual cycle

The anterior pituitary gland (under the control of the hypothalamus) and the ovary are the endocrine glands involved with hormonal activity during the menstrual cycle.

Secretions of the anterior pituitary gland
- *Follicle stimulating hormone (FSH)* ripens the graafian follicle
- *Luteinising hormone (LH)* maintains the corpus luteum
- *Prolactin* begins early preparation of the breasts for the function of lactation.

Secretions of the ovary
- *Oestrogen* is essential for the development of female characteristics. It produces re-growth of the endometrium
- *Progesterone* is indispensable since it stimulates necessary physiological preparations for pregnancy
- *Relaxin* ripens the follicle and allows it to rupture.

On Day 1   Taking Day 1 of a 28-day menstrual cycle as the day menstrual bleeding commences, oestrogen levels in the woman's circulatory system are low but the stimulus of follicle stimulating hormone is maximal. The function of FSH is to develop the graafian follicles by increasing the follicular fluid and granulosa cells and thus increasing the secretion of oestrogen.

By Day 5,   when the shedding of the endometrium is complete, oestrogen levels are rising and begin to produce new growth and proliferation of the endometrium. The theca interna cells are producing oestrogen at this time and, in addition to endometrial growth, stroma cells increase and spiral arterioles lengthen.

After Day 8   development of the graafian follicle is no longer dependent upon the pituitary secretion of FSH, and the level of this hormone begins to decrease. The graafian follicle continues to produce its own oestrogen from the theca cells and the levels of oestrogen continue to rise. Some fluid and sodium retention in the body tissues, especially in the endometrium, is brought about by this rise. At an unknown point in this ascending scale of oestrogen level, FSH is inhibited and luteinising hormone released. LH now influences the last stage of graafian follicle maturation. Relaxin changes the walls of the follicle and allows the ovum to escape. **Ovulation thus occurs on the 14th day of a 28-day cycle** but its timing varies with the length of each individual cycle.

The effect of increased oestrogen secretion is to act now on the cervical mucus. The glands secrete more of it and it is much less tenacious. As this is the time for optimum fertilisation, the spermatozoa are aided on their way into the female genital tract by this cervical fluid.

It is of interest to note here that, while LH acts in conjunction with FSH to effect ovulation, research has demonstrated that it cannot function unless FSH has preceded it.

The post-ovulatory phase is always of 14 days duration since LH is only functional for that period.

Following ovulation there is a drop in oestrogen levels and in some women this produces slight endometrial bleeding (spotting) – withdrawal bleeding. The granulosa cells, however, continue to secrete oestrogen. The corpus luteum begins to hypertrophy and to secrete increasing amounts of progesterone and relaxin. At the time of ovulation, due to the surge of progesterone, there is a slight rise in body temperature. Other side-effects are described later in this chapter.

In the endometrium, there is an increased fluid and sodium retention, higher than that which was caused by oestrogen in the first phase of the cycle. Secretory glands become more active and blood vessels, influenced by relaxin, are capable of carrying an increased blood supply. Glucose is laid down and there is continued growth of endometrium, also influenced by relaxin.

Prolactin is discovered in the urine of women during this phase and it is believed that LH cannot fulfil its function unless prolactin is present. This hormone also stimulates development of mammary tissue and secretory activity.

Day 25–26 The corpus luteum begins to degenerate (unless the ovum has been fertilised) because the pituitary withdraws LH. Levels of both oestrogen and progesterone are consequently reduced and preparations of the uterus to receive a fertilised ovum cease.

On Day 28 The regenerated and secretory endometrium is shed. But, as LH is withdrawn, the body prepares for pregnancy once again with the release of FSH.

This cycle will continue for 35 years or more if the menarche is commenced at the average age of 12. Over 400 ova will be produced. The cycle ceases during pregnancy as further hormonal influences play their part and the menstrual cycle and ovulation can be suppressed if hormonal methods of contraception are practised.

The cyclical syndrome

The changes in hormone balance which occur during the menstrual cycle inevitably cause changes throughout the body. To some extent, the early signs and symptoms of pregnancy are experienced during the second half of the cycle, but to the majority of women these are only transitory discomforts accepted as being inevitable and medical advice is rarely sought, or, indeed, needed. The most common symptoms experienced are:

- Enlargement and tenderness of breasts and nipples
- Fluid in the breast
- Digestive disturbances, e.g. epigastric discomfort, heartburn and constipation
- Increased frequency of micturition
- Increased amount of vaginal discharge
- Increased activity of the skin
- Weight gain.

These conditions are largely brought about by the relaxation of smooth muscle caused by progesterone. Proliferation of tissues in the breast and genital tract, resulting from hormonal influence, accounts for the symptoms experienced directly there. Retention of mineral salts leads to retention of body fluid, causing oedema and weight gain. This is probably the causative factor of headaches and visual disturbances. Some women actually become sleepy and inert, probably due to deposits of glucose in the uterine lining.

During the secretory phase it has become an established fact that judgement is impaired. Careless mistakes are made, women are more accident prone, and the behaviour of schoolgirls is said to worsen.

The majority of women accept all these things as inevitable – they probably do not even think about them – and are certainly not incapacitated by them. A minority present with more severe symptoms which they cannot control. Due to less well-balanced endocrine activity, they complain of nervous tension, irritability, depression and are generally difficult to live with. These women should be advised to seek medical advice if their symptoms do not abate; treatment lies in a combination of reassurance, controlled diet and drugs. Low salt intake and diuretics are used to combat fluid retention and oedema, adequate roughage in the diet and aperients to treat constipation. Tranquillising drugs reduce the degree of irritability and depression is counteracted with drugs of the stimulant group.

It is also worth remembering that conditions such as asthma, migraine and epilepsy are sometimes exacerbated in the secretory phase of the menstrual cycle and, if this is so, a similar exacerbation should be watched for during pregnancy.

REVISION QUESTIONS

What is an endocrine gland?

Name the four phases of the menstrual cycle.

Which hormone is directly responsible for the production of oestrogen?

Where is oestrogen produced?

At which stage of the menstrual cycle is oestrogen at its peak?

Where is the corpus luteum and what hormone does it produce?

What effect does progesterone have on involuntary (smooth or unstriped) muscle?

How can levels of oestrogen and progesterone be assessed?

Why does ovulation occur before the lining of the uterus is at its thickest and most vascular?

Suggest how ovulation may be prevented by the administration of a hormone.

Describe the pathway through which the fertilised egg passes in order to reach the uterus. What may happen if anything obstructs the passage of the fertilised egg into the uterus?

Describe the structure of the ovary. What hormones does it produce and what influence do they have on the course of pregnancy?

Describe the anatomy and physiology of the ovaries.

What is a hormone? Describe the menstrual cycle, paying particular attention to the controlling role of hormones in its regulation.

At which time in the menstrual cycle is pregnancy a) most likely b) least likely to occur? Show how pregnancy may be prevented by the administration of a hormone.

Draw a diagram to show the relationship during the menstrual cycle between ovulation, the thickness of the endometrium and the concentration of oestrogen and progesterone in the bloodstream.

REFERENCES AND FURTHER READING

Books and reports

Carpenter M 1986 Curing PMT. Century Arrow, London

Dalton K 1969 The menstrual cycle. Penguin, Harmondsworth

Dalton K 1979 Once a month: the menstrual syndrome, its causes and consequences. Harvester Press, Hassocks

Shreeve C 1983 The pre-menstrual syndrome: the curse that can be cured. Thorsons Press, Wellingborough

Wilson E W 1976 The menstrual cycle. Lloyd Luke, London

Articles

Gondos B et al 1986 Onset of oogenesis in the fetal human ovary. American Journal of Obstetrics and Gynecology 155: 189

Research review 1982 The pre-menstrual syndrome. IPPF Research in Reproduction (Jan) 1

10 The male reproductive system

The organs of the male reproductive tract are derived from the same embryonic tissue as those of the female reproductive tract. The development or repressed growth of particular cells is determined by the XX or XY chromosome pattern at the time of fertilisation. For instance, it was noted in Chapters 4 and 5 that the urethral crypts and ducts of the female are rudimentary analogues of the male prostate gland while the glans and body of the female clitoris are analogous to the male penis.

Like the female reproductive system, the male has both internal and external organs of reproduction (Fig. 10.1)

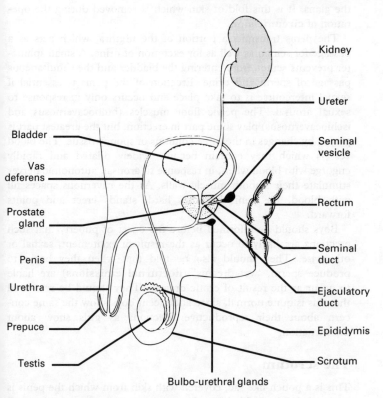

Fig. 10.1 Male organs of reproduction.

External organs
1. The *penis*, which transmits the urethra
2. The *scrotum*, which contains:
   - the *testes*
   - the *epididymis*
   - part of the *vas deferens*.

Internal organs
- The remainder of the *vas deferens*
- The *seminal vesicles* and *ducts*
- The *ejaculatory ducts*
- The *prostate gland*
- The *bulbo-urethral* (or *Cowper's*) *glands*.

The penis

For most of the time the penis hangs flaccidly, suspended between the thighs, hanging downwards in front of the scrotal sac. It is expanded at the distal end to form an acorn-shaped structure, the **glans penis**. The penis is composed of three columns of sponge-like erectile tissue with a rich blood supply. This is enclosed in a firm sheath of fibrous tissue and is covered with skin which is continuous with that of the scrotum and groins. The skin covering the glans penis is doubled back on itself to form the **prepuce or fore-skin**, except in young infants, where the prepuce is still attached to the glans. It is this fold of skin which is removed during the operation of **circumcision**.

The penis transmits a portion of the urethra, which acts as a passage for semen as well as for excretion of urine. A small sphincter prevents semen from entering the bladder and the simultaneous passage of sperm and urine. Erection of the penis is essential if sexual intercourse is to take place and occurs only in response to sexual arousal. The pelvic floor muscles (bulbocavernosus and ischiocavernosus) play some part in erection, but the greatest part is played by changes in the three columns of spongy tissue. The blood vessels which they contain become widely dilated and rapidly engorge with blood when, in response to arousal, autonomic nerves stimulate their smooth muscle walls. As the cavernous spaces fill with blood, the penis becomes hard, stands erect and points forward.

Boys should be informed before the onset of puberty that such erections are likely to occur as the result of excitement, sexual or otherwise. They should also be told that when they begin to produce sperm, 'wet dreams' (**nocturnal emissions**) are liable to occur as the result of erotic dreams. They should be reassured that this is quite normal, since adolescent boys show the same concern about their reproductive functions as girls show about menstruation.

The scrotum

This is a pouch-like sac, covered with skin from which the penis is suspended. It is divided by a fibrous septum into two cavities each of which contain a testis, an epididymis and the initial portion of the vas deferens. The scrotum contains no subcutaneous fat but has muscle tissue which can retract the testicles in order to protect them from trauma.

The testes (or testicles)

These are formed in the fetal abdomen about the 28th week of intrauterine life and descend into the scrotum to be supported by the spermatic cord before birth. Failure of the testes to descend is known as **cryptorchism** and is a cause of male infertility, because sperm production requires a temperature below that of normal body heat. The testes do not function fully until stimulated by the anterior pituitary gland at puberty.

Size, shape and appearance　In appearance, the testes are oval structures, white in colour, about 4 cm long, 2.5 cm wide and 3 cm thick. They each weigh between 10 and 14 g.

Gross structure　The testes are enclosed in a protective fibrous capsule, the **tunica albuginea**, and are covered by a serous membrane, the **tunica vaginalis,** which enables each testis to move freely within its scrotal cavity.

Microscopic structure　The glandular tissue composing each testis is divided into 200–300 lobes. Each lobe contains convoluted seminiferous tubules which empty into the vas deferens.

Seminiferous tubules start to develop from syncytial cells when the boy is about 7 years old and progressive development occurs until the age of 16 when the testes reach adult size. The tubules are lined with a basal layer of connective tissue on which lies **germinal epithelium** from which the sperm are produced after puberty.

On microscopic examination an occasional **spermatogonia** may be seen before the boy is 11 years old but the production of sperm in any number or degree of maturity does not usually occur until a boy is at least 12. Production of mature sperm rarely occurs before he is 16.

Sertoli cells develop at the same time as germinal epithelium and nourish the spermatozoa throughout their development in the testes. **Interstitial cells** develop at the same time but more slowly than the seminiferous tubules. They produce testosterone and are not completely developed until the boy is about 18 years of age.

Functions　The testes have two functions:

1. *To produce testosterone*, the hormone which controls secondary male characteristics
2. *To produce spermatozoa.*

The functions of the testes can be affected by **orchitis**, which can result from mumps or other acute infections. Such an infection can result in failure of the testes to produce spermatozoa.

Epididymis (*pl.* epididymides)

These are fine convoluted tubules, each about 6 metres in length, which connect the testes and the vasa deferentia. The tubules have a ciliated epithelial lining which helps the sperm to migrate to the vas deferens.

Vas deferens (*pl.* vasa deferentia)

These are tubes, each about 45 cm in length, which convey spermatozoa from the epididymides to the prostatic urethra. Unlike the epididymis, the vas deferens has no ciliated lining since the secretions of the seminal vesicles and prostate gland provide a medium to aid the passage of spermatozoa. Sperm are stored in the vasa while they mature and increase their motility.

The vasa deferentia are the structures which are ligated or cut during vasectomy. Sperm are still produced and enter the vas but they cannot be ejaculated and so degenerate.

Seminal vesicles

These are small, irregularly-shaped sacs about 5 cm long lying between the base of the bladder and the rectum. Their function is to secrete a thick, yellowish-coloured fluid which is added to the sperm to form seminal fluid. It contains glucose and other substances to nourish the sperm. Each vesicle opens into a **seminal duct** which joins the vas deferens on the corresponding side to form the **ejaculatory duct**.

Ejaculatory ducts

Each duct is formed by the union of the vas deferens and the seminal duct. The ejaculatory ducts are approximately 2.5 cm long. They pass through the **prostate gland** and join the urethra. So, in effect, they connect the vasa deferentia and urethra.

Prostate gland

A cone-shaped structure 4 cm long, 3 cm wide, 2 cm deep, weighing about 8 g, the prostate surrounds the upper part of the urethra and lies in direct contact with the neck of the bladder. It is composed of glandular tissue and involuntary muscle fibres and is enclosed in a fibrous capsule.

The muscle tissue of the gland aids in ejaculation.

Prostatic secretion is being constantly manufactured and is excreted in the urine. About 1 ml is produced each day but the amount is dependent upon testosterone levels since it is that hormone which stimulates secretion. It has a pH of 6.6 and is similar in composition to plasma but contains additional constituents such as cholesterol, citric acid and hyaluronidase, an enzyme. Prostatic secretion is added to the sperm and seminal fluid as they pass into the urethra.

The prostate gland quite commonly becomes enlarged in middle-aged and elderly men and this, or any other pressure on the urethral sphincter or the urethra itself, results in acute retention of urine. The condition is relieved by passing a catheter into the bladder or by prostatectomy in suitable patients.

Bulbo-urethral (Cowper's) glands

Small glands about the size of a pea, yellow in colour, lying just below the prostate gland. Their ducts, about 3 cm long, open into the urethra before it reaches the penile portion. Secretions from the glands are added to the **seminal fluid**. The bulbo-urethral glands release a small amount of fluid prior to ejaculation and this lubricates the penis, facilitating its entry into the vagina.

While the prostatic secretion alone has a pH of 6.6, the pH of seminal fluid as a whole is the same as that of blood, 7.5.

Seminal fluid

This is the fluid in which the spermatozoa are suspended. It nourishes them and aids their motility. Passing from the seminal vesicles and ducts, it travels through the ejaculatory ducts to the urethra where prostatic secretions and secretions from the bulbo-urethral glands are added. It is finally ejaculated during sexual excitement. The prostatic secretion is the largest component of seminal fluid.

PRODUCTION AND PASSAGE OF SPERMATOZOA (Fig. 10.2)

Production

Full spermatogenesis is achieved in most males by their 16th year and then continues throughout life. It does not occur simultaneously in all seminiferous tubules or even in different parts of the same tubule. The cycle commences in the basal layer of germinal epithelium in response to the follicle stimulating hormone. As the spermatozoa develop they rise nearer to the lumen of the tubule. They take about 10 days to mature.

Spermatogonia

These are the primitive structures and reproduce by mitosis at least once. Following reproduction they are nourished by Sertoli cells and develop into primary spermatocytes.

Primary spermatocytes

These contain the **diploid** number of chromosomes in their nuclei and undergo meiosis (reduction division and interchange of genetic material). One spermatocyte produces two daughter cells, the secondary spermatocytes.

Secondary spermatocytes

These **haploid** cells now undergo a second meiotic division in order to make further re-arrangement of genetic material. The in-

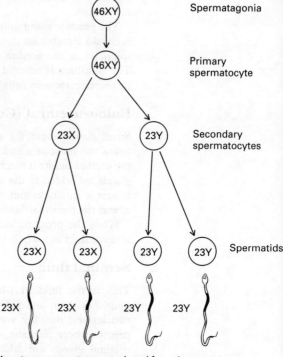

Fig. 10.2 Production of spermatozoa.

4 mature spermatozoa produced from 1 spermatocyte

fluence of luteinising hormone (LH) is necessary for the next stages of development.

Spermatids These are the cells produced by the second meiotic division. Nourished by the Sertoli cells, the largest part of the spermatid containing the nucleus becomes the *head* of the mature spermatozoon.

Mature spermatozoon *Four* mature spermatozoa have thus developed from one original spermatogonia. Two spermatozoa will carry an 'X' female-determining chromosome. When one of these sperm unites with an ovum, the normal human somatic pattern of 23 paired cells will be restored. The mature sperm consists of:

1. *A head* which not only contains the nucleus with its chromosomes and genetic material but is covered by an **acrosome**. The latter contains **hyaluronidase**, the enzyme which facilitates fertilisation of the ovum (see Ch. 12)
2. *A neck* which unites the head to the body
3. *A body* which is concerned with the production of energy, required for motility
4. *A tail* whose lashing movements propel the sperm into the vas deferens and ejaculatory ducts.

During spermatogenesis the primary spermatocyte reproduces to produce two secondary spermatocytes and these in turn produce four equally-sized spermatozoa. The outcome of oogenesis is quite different. The primary oocyte produces **one** secondary oocyte and one polar body. The secondary oocyte and the first polar body give rise to **one** mature ovum and three polar bodies. The three polar bodies normally degenerate.

It is also of interest to note that while the mature spermatozoa is the smallest cell in the body, the ovum is the largest (see Ch. 9, p. 140).

In the female, the sex chromosomes are homogenous and are called XX. The male carries dissimilar (heterogenous) sex-determining chromosomes, one being an X, a female determining cell. The smaller of the pair is a Y, a male-determining cell.

Normal semen analysis

Average amount of ejaculate is 3.5 ml but the normal range lies between 2 and 6 ml.

Average density is 60–150 000 000 sperm per millilitre of seminal fluid. Of these 75% are mobile and 20–25% will be malformed in some way.

Rate of movement varies with the pH of environmental fluid. A speed of 2–3 mm per minute is the average but this slows considerable to about 0.5 mm per minute in the acid vaginal secretion.

Content Seminal fluid is made up largely of prostatic secretion but secretion of the seminal vesicles and Cowper's glands all help to nourish as well as provide means of transport for the sperm. The alkaline medium and the hyaluronidase content are both important factors. In particular, hyaluronidase aids the passage through the tenacious cervical mucus as well as assisting in the breakdown of the protective protoplasm that surrounds the ovum, thereby facilitating fertilisation.

Pathway of spermatozoa

At first the spermatozoa have little motility of their own and need fluid secretions in which to move. From the **seminiferous tubules** they pass to the **epididymides** where they remain for some time. Their movement is aided by the ciliated epithelial lining and they reach the **vas deferens**. The secretions of the seminal vesicles are added in the vas deferens which further aids sperm motility and they pass through the **ejaculatory duct** and the **prostate** gland where prostatic secretions are added. Much more mobile now, they reach the urethra where secretions of the bulbo-urethral gland are mixed with the seminal fluid. They are **finally ejaculated** during sexual excitement and only become freely mobile when **deposited in the vagina**. Their pathway now lies through the cervix and the **uterus** to the **fallopian tube**.

To sum up the pathway:

- seminiferous tubules
- epididymis
- vas deferens
- ejaculatory duct
- prostate gland
- urethra and ejaculation

- vagina
- cervix
- uterus
- fallopian tube and fertilisation.

REVISION QUESTIONS

Draw a large, fully labelled diagram to illustrate and explain the organs of the male reproductive system.

Write a detailed account of the production, storage and passage of spermatozoa.

Describe the structure and functions of the testes. What conditions might result in male sterility?

Describe the following conditions:

1. Cryptorchism
2. Orchitis
3. Hypospadias
4. Phimosis.

For what reasons might the operation of circumcision be carried out? What structures are involved?

REFERENCES AND FURTHER READING

Books and reports
Llewellyn-Jones D 1987 Everyman. Oxford University Press, Oxford
McKee L, O'Brien M 1982 The father figure. Tavistock Publications, London
Seel R 1987 The uncertain father: exploring modern fatherhood. Gateway Books, Bath

Articles
Alibhai Y 1988 Trouble and strife: what happens when the old Adam becomes a new father. New State and Society (Nov): 22–23
Bedford V A, Johnson N 1988 The role of the father. Midwifery 4: 190–195
Benuevenati P et al 1989 Psychological and psychophysiological problems of fatherhood. Journal of Psychology, Obstetrics and Gynaecology 10 (suppl 2): 35–41
Donaldson J 1991 Facing up to fatherhood. Parents (Jan): 66–68
Jordan P, Wall V 1990 Breast feeding and fathers. Birth 17(4): 210–213
Purves L 1990 What are fathers for? Parents (June): 34–35

11 Conception, contraception, infertility

CONCEPTION

The optimum time for a pregnancy to be initiated is within 24 hours of ovulation. Intercourse during the 24 hours preceding ovulation will supply sperms to the fallopian tubes, ready for the appearance of the ovum. It is therefore important to each woman trying to conceive that she know the approximate date of ovulation.

The following methods can be used to assess the date of ovulation.

1. Calendar method Records should be kept over a period of at least 6 months, charting the first day of each menstrual period (Day 1 of the menstrual flow) and thus calculating the time of ovulation – 15 days prior to that particular period. In this way the days of successive months when a woman is likely to start menstruating, and therefore the days when she is likely to ovulate, can be estimated. If the menses are irregular, such calculation is impossible.

Even when the cycle is as regular as clockwork, it must be borne in mind that the pituitary gland which directs the menstrual cycle is actually itself under the influence of the hypothalamus and therefore emotional and physical factors such as a family row, or death, or a new job, or moving house, or even a holiday abroad may upset the 'clockwork'.

It is therefore usual, and more accurate, to use this method in association with one or both of the following methods.

2. Temperature method It is now recognised that the release of progesterone results in a rise of body temperature of up to 0.5°C. The temperature drops a little immediately before ovulation and then rises immediately afterwards. This system therefore requires the recording of the oral temperature immediately upon waking each morning. (Family Planning Clinics will supply both charts and thermometers.) The rise must be sustained for 24 hours in order for ovulation to be confirmed. Used alone, this method may be misleading, since a rise of temperature can denote infection and a lower temperature sometimes results from drugs such as aspirin.

3. Changes in cervical mucus The rising oestrogen level just prior to ovulation produces an increase in cervical secretion as well as reducing its viscosity. This aids the passage of spermatozoa and has already been described on page 144. As the secretion becomes part of vaginal secretions, its change can be recognised by the woman who hopes to conceive. Nevertheless it may take 2 or 3 months for partners who have not previously recognised its significance to become aware of it.

A more vague symptom of ovulation is Mittelschmerz, the lower abdominal pain which occurs with rupture of the follicle, as the fallopian tubes increase their peristaltic action. But this, taken by itself, is not a reliable indication.

Most women, of course, become pregnant without difficulty. This would be early advice given to couples who are concerned because a pregnancy has not occurred.

CONTRACEPTION

'Natural' methods

Safe period

This is a very misleading term. The name is wrongfully applied because the method is not a very reliable way of avoiding pregnancy. Its safety lies in eliciting the date of ovulation and then avoiding intercourse at that time. The couple need to remember that the lifespan of the ovum is approximately 48 hours but that sperm, once inside the uterus, can survive for up to 5 days. When considering the safe period as a method of contraception it is therefore advisable to leave a 5-day margin when intercourse must be avoided on each side of the 48 hours following the expected date of ovulation. Therefore, presuming that the menstrual cycle is an average one of 28 days, intercourse should be avoided between the 10th and 18th days inclusively. The greatest problem is to elicit the actual time of ovulation.

Coitus interruptus

Like the safe period, this method is only considered when the usual contraceptive devices are not acceptable. Neither partner is able to achieve complete sexual satisfaction and theoretically the technique can only result in physical and mental tension. Harmonious relationships must be difficult to maintain by this method, as indeed by complete abstinence from intercourse, and both these methods should be considered harmful if used in the long term.

Some research has shown, however, that where coitus interruptus is used by married couples it does not appear to cause any marital tension and the method must therefore be included here. For some people it does seem to work, and is probably better than nothing in an emergency situation! Coitus interruptus does *not* have a 100% failure rate!

Changes in cervical mucus

An increase in the amount and viscosity of cervical secretions, as described above, indicates days when there should be abstinence from intercourse if pregnancy is to be avoided.

Mechanical methods

Condoms A condom, made of thin but strong vulcanised latex, can be worn by the male to prevent seminal fluid from entering the vagina, but it sometimes has disadvantages (Fig. 11.1A). Some men find it bothersome to use, to others it causes irritation and lack of potency, while many partners complain that it is messy and reduces the pleasure of intimate contact. It is one of the more reliable methods of contraception, although there is always the possibility that the sheath may rupture or become dislodged during intercourse. For this reason the female partner should use one of the chemical spermicidal preparations when her partner uses a sheath.

The failure rates are high in the very young, possibly because there is genital contact before the condom is put on or because withdrawal is delayed until the penis is quite flaccid and the condom may 'leak' semen when being removed. Some 'fun' condoms do not conform to BSI standards and there is a greater risk that they may rupture during intercourse. Possibly the condom's greatest advantage is that, while it offers no protection against herpes, it does offer protection against other sexually-transmitted diseases, including carcinoma of the cervix.

Because of the increasing awareness of AIDS, new, condom-like devices for females are currently being manufactured and tested in Europe and the USA. One variety has undergone a pilot study in this country and has proved acceptable to users. A larger study has now been completed to test its contraceptive reliability and the condom is now available in the UK.

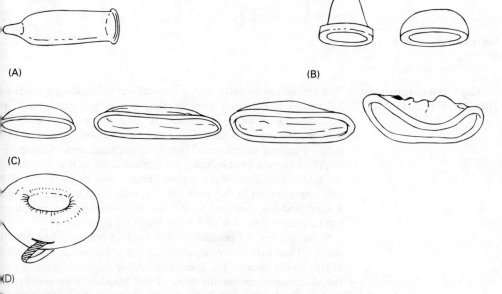

Fig. 11.1 Mechanical methods of contraception. (A) Male condom (B) Cervical caps (C) Diaphragms (D) Vaginal sponge.

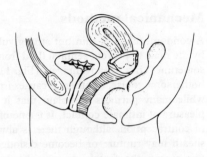

Fig. 11.2 Cervical cap in place.

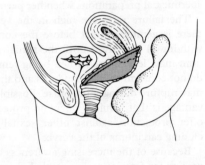

Fig. 11.3 Vaginal diaphragm in place.

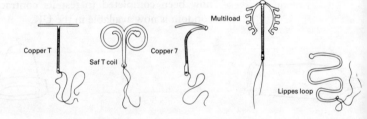

Copper T

Saf T coil

Copper 7

Multiload

Lippes loop

Fig. 11.4 Intra-uterine devices.

Caps and diaphragms
(Figs 11.1B & C, 11.2, 11.3)

The female can be fitted with a cervical cap or diaphragm made of vulcanised latex which fits completely over the cervix and so occludes the entrance to the uterus. Both come in a variety of designs and sizes and should be fitted by a person fully trained in family planning techniques. Their function, regardless of design, is to prevent sperm from entering the cervical canal so that they die in the acid environment of the vagina. Because they may not provide a 100% sperm-tight fit they must, like the male condom, be used with a spermicidal preparation to increase their effectiveness and must not be removed for at least 8 hours following intercourse.

Some women do not favour this method because they find it messy. They may suffer vaginal irritation as the result of a minor allergy to the latex or the spermicide. Also, due to the pressure of the diaphragm rim on the base of the bladder, a proportion of women develop urinary tract infections.

Although, unlike the condom, the insertion of a diaphragm can be independent of intercourse it is not disposable and requires washing, drying and inspection after use. With the advent of the contraceptive pill, caps and diaphragms fell out of favour but they do appear to be becoming more popular again. They require practice to be used correctly but, on the whole, they do not cause so many side-effects.

Contraceptive sponge
(Fig. 11.1D)

These disposable sponges have a small 'dimple' in the centre which is meant to fit over the cervical os. A tape is attached to the sponge to aid its removal. Impregnated with spermicide, the sponge is moistened with water before being inserted high into the vagina. It can be placed in position up to 24 hours before intercourse and should be left in situ for 6 hours afterwards.

The sponge does not really have any advantage over spermicides used by themselves and the failure rate is higher than that of the diaphragm used with a spermicide.

Chemical products
(spermicides)

These are manufactured in the form of vaginal pessaries, creams, pastes and jellies. They act partly by forming a barrier against the sperm and partly by destroying the sperm by their chemical action. Used alone they are not wholly reliable and are of greater benefit when used in conjunction with male or female mechanical appliances. New chemicals are currently being studied which use better base materials and alter the cervical mucus so that sperm are destroyed. The most recent inhibits the action of the sperms' own enzymes so that fertilisation is not possible.

Intrauterine devices
(IUDs; Fig. 11.4)

These are solid objects which, when placed in the uterine cavity, cause changes in the uterine endometrium which render it hostile to the embedding ovum. They do not prevent ovulation. They can also be inserted within a 5-day period after ovulation if there is any possibility that unwanted fertilisation occurred at that time. They come in various shapes and sizes but most are made of a plastic or silicone material, some have a copper-bearing wire and some release hormones. *Copper*: is toxic to the sperm and to the blastocyst; *hormone-releasing* IUDs release progesterone or progestogens and deter the sperm in their attempts to penetrate the cervix and the uterus.

All IUDs have a tape or marker thread by which the woman can be reassured that the IUD has not been expelled from the uterus. It also aids removal of the device when it needs to be changed or when it is no longer required.

Currently being studied are hormone-bearing vaginal rings which release their chemicals into the vaginal mucosa. They can be removed for intercourse. All intrauterine devices are highly effective.

The disadvantage of this particular method lies in the fact that the device may be unknowingly expelled by the wearer and that pregnancy may occur through no faulty technique of her own. There is also a risk of ectopic pregnancy.

Some women find the intrauterine device unacceptable because for them it produces excessive menstrual bleeding and uterine cramps.

The contraceptive 'pill'

The surest way of preventing pregnancy is for the female partner to take the contraceptive 'pill'. There are several types of this pill but they each contain carefully balanced oestrogen/progesterone hormones which inhibit ovulation. The pill is prescribed only under strict medical supervision and is controlled by Schedule 4 of the Drugs Act. To be fully effective the pills must be taken exactly as the instructions state.

Some women suffer from mild but unpleasant side-effects and this method is not acceptable to them.

Three types of pill are currently available.

1. Combined oral contraceptive

These contain 30–50 µg of oestrogen and between 0.5 and 2 mg of progestogen (norethisterone). Oestrogen suppresses ovulation and progesterone is added for cycle control. Their objective is to prevent maturation of the graafian follicle and formation of the corpus luteum. These contraceptive combinations also:

- Render the cervical mucus impenetrable to sperm by increasing its viscosity
- Reduce the motility of the fallopian tubes, thereby reducing peristaltic action so that the surviving sperm find it very difficult to move along them to the uterus.

The menstrual cycle is suppressed but cyclical, withdrawal bleeding occurs when the daily pill is replaced by a placebo.

It is possible to produce a regimen (triphasic combined pill) which produces 1 week of bleeding every 12 weeks, but most women favour the monthly cycle.

The method is highly acceptable since it reduces cyclical disorders and is aesthetically acceptable, as it is not associated with the act of intercourse.

It does however have disadvantages, having side-effects such as hypertension, deep venous thrombosis, pulmonary embolism, myocardial infarction and cerebrovascular accident. Consequently, its use is not now advised for women over 35, heavy smokers or those who are obese. Those with a history of cardiovascular disease would also not be considered as suitable subjects.

More recently, to lessen the incidence of side-effects, pills containing only 20–30 µg of oestrogen have been introduced but there is an increased risk of pregnancy if even one pill is missed.

2. Progestogen only pill

These are completely oestrogen free and have a varied effect on ovulation, in some women suppressing it completely. In others, the follicle ripens normally but there is a shortened luteal phase and no production of progesterone. In some women, ultrasound scans have shown ovaries with abnormal follicles.

The efficacy of these drugs is dependent upon a very strict regime. The pill must be taken at the same time every day and it is extremely important that no pill is omitted. If taken only 3 hours late, extra contraceptive measures must be used during the next 48 hours. It is imperative that the instructions are followed implicitly if pregnancy is to be avoided.

The contraceptive action of the progestogen-only pill lies in its action on the cervical mucus, making it tenacious and hostile to sperm, and in reducing peristaltic action of the fallopian tubes so that sperm which do survive find it extremely difficult or impossible to reach the uterus.

They are used mostly for women over 35, those with diabetes or those with a history of thromboembolic disease or hypertension. They are also suitable for the woman who is breast feeding. It is important that the women for whom they are prescribed are intelligent enough to recognise the importance of the strict regime and yet do not have an obsessional neurosis about it.

3. Sequentials   Sequentials are very rarely prescribed now in the UK. Oestrogen only is contained in the pills taken during the first half of the cycle and then, during the second half, both oestrogen and progesterone. The effect of this balance of hormones is to suppress ovulation and, because the oestrogen level is so high, it will also suppress lactation if given to a postnatal patient. Sequentials produce many side-effects, including weight gain, breast changes, nausea, headaches and loss of libido.

4. Depot contraceptives   These contraceptive measures are administered by intramuscular injection and are progestogenic steroids.

Depo-Provera (DMPA): an injection of 150 mg is administered every 12 weeks.

Noristerat (NET): an injection of 200 mg is given every 8 weeks.

These methods are more effective than any other in use, although they do have a marginally higher rate of failure in younger women. Their greatest advantage lies in the fact that the woman cannot forget to take them. They do not affect lactation in the breast feeding woman and may even increase the supply.

For women who are awaiting sterilisation or whose husbands have recently had a vasectomy they are invaluable, as they are also for women of low intelligence who cannot be relied upon to use other contraceptive methods meticulously.

In the presence of sickle-cell disease, this contraceptive measure appears to bring about an improvement in the woman's condition, although the mechanism is not understood.

The disadvantages are a delay in the return of fertility, menstrual chaos in some women, excessive weight gain and a possible recurrence of enuresis from earlier years.

Resumption of oral contraceptives   Following delivery it is usual for the postnatal mother to resume her oral contraceptives on Day 21 following delivery.

The role of the midwife

Unless the midwife is a trained and experienced family-planning counsellor, her main role is one of referral to the appropriate clinic or general practitioner's surgery.

General, careless remarks are best avoided, for it is of the greatest importance that only accurate advice should be given pertaining to each individual woman and that only sound literature is displayed. There are common misunderstandings, for instance, regarding:

- The 'safe' period
- Heavy petting
- Coitus interruptus
- Use of the condom
- The safety of spermicides alone
- Removal of the diaphragm.

Other misunderstandings relate to:

- Day 1 of the menstrual cycle
- The 'missing' of a contraceptive pill
- Observing a regular time of day at which the contraceptive pill is taken
- Safety of the pill during bouts of sickness
- The availability of postcoital contraception
- Resumption of the contraceptive pill on Day 21 following delivery.

The midwife should remember, too, that contraceptive advice is not sought by many women because they regard it as offensive for ethnic, ethical, cultural or religious reasons.

Female sterilisation

When further pregnancies are likely to endanger a woman's health and well-being, or if family-planning methods have been unsuccessful in limiting the number of her pregnancies, some obstetricians will offer the opportunity of sterilisation. Here again, the offer should be made tentatively since, like contraception, the idea is not acceptable to all women.

The method most commonly used today is sealing of the fallopian tubes with bipolar diathermy so that the lumen is occluded. The operation is carried out by means of laparoscopy and the woman is normally discharged 24 hours later.

If this method is either not suitable or not available, the tubes are bisected, a small portion is removed and the ends are then ligated and/or buried. Alternatively, clips or rings may be used to occlude the lumen.

If the operation is to be carried out postnatally it is usually delayed until after the postnatal examination in order to reduce the risks of haemorrhage and infection.

Sterilisation should be regarded as the ultimate means of preventing pregnancy because reconstitution of the tubes in a reversal process does not have a very high success rate.

Male sterilisation

The operation of vasectomy involves sealing, ligating or bisecting the vas deferens. Spermatozoa are still produced, of course, but they cannot be ejaculated because their pathway is obstructed. The operation can be carried out in a day hospital.

A period of 12 weeks should then be allowed to elapse before the man can be considered sterile because spermatozoa will be present in the vas at the time of surgery. When a specimen of his seminal fluid is pronounced sperm-free by the laboratory, his sterility is confirmed. The need to use a contraceptive until the time of such confirmation must be stressed to both partners. Many general practitioners will offer the female partner the choice of an 'injectable' contraceptive.

INFERTILITY

About 10% of married couples seek medical advice regarding infertility when, after 2 years of married life, they find that they are still childless. Investigations must always commence with enquiries into their general health and way of life and a careful medical history must be taken. Tactful enquiries should also elicit that the marriage has actually been consummated and that they are sexually active. Where sexual problems exist, psychosexual counselling and education is advisable and a couple should be referred to the appropriate clinics. Details of **menstrual history** are essential. It is necessary to know if the cycle is regular and whether conception has ever occurred. If the woman did conceive, then was her pregnancy spontaneously, therapeutically or otherwise terminated? As a result of informal conversation during the interview, it should also be possible to assess the degree of anxiety which exists. This, in itself, is often a real obstruction to conception.

Causes of female infertility

Hormonal

Disorders of the pituitary, thyroid, adrenal glands or ovaries causing:

1. Failure to ovulate
2. Failure of uterine endometrium to become proliferative and secretory
3. Vaginal or cervical secretions which are unfavourable to sperm
4. A failure in motility of the fallopian tubes which prevents spermatozoa from reaching the uterus.

It is now recognised that abnormalities in the luteal phase of the menstrual cycle are an important cause of infertility. All appears to be well, but when hormone levels are assessed over the whole menstrual cycle, the **rate of progesterone secretion** as well as its **highest peak** is much **lower** than in fertile women.

Hormone levels can be assessed:

- In samples of intravenous blood and urine
- By histology of vaginal epithelium and uterine endometrium.

Ovulation can be confirmed by:

- Calendar, cervical mucus and body temperature methods (see p. 155 ff.)
- Ovulation prediction test – on sale at chemists' shops
- Ultrasound examination, which will reveal any ripening follicles. If the woman is found to be not ovulating then, under strict medical supervision, ovulation can be induced by carefully calculated doses of clomiphene, menotrophin or other gonadotrophic hormones
- Uterine endometrium can be obtained by dilatation and curettage and histology studies undertaken in the laboratory.

Obstruction   Obstructed fallopian tubes account for about one-third of the causes of infertility. The obstruction may be caused by:

1. *Congenital defect*
2. *General pelvic inflammatory disease*, e.g. appendicitis and peritonitis
3. *An ascending genital tract infection*, e.g. gonorrhoea.

The tubes can be examined by laparoscopy following the injection of a dye into the uterine cavity which then overspills into the peritoneal cavity, or by insufflation. In many instances the blockage is removed by these investigations and many women conceive soon afterwards. If a hysterosalpingogram and X-ray is used, the position of the obstruction can be demonstrated.

Simultaneously the ovaries can be examined at laparoscopy for the presence of ripening graafian follicles or a corpus luteum.

The presence of pelvic infection would be evident also.

Where a tube remains persistently obstructed, there might be a possibility of its being reconstituted by microsurgery but current results show that only one-third of all patients who undergo surgery subsequently become pregnant. Efforts are being made to improve microsurgery and to 'transplant' tubes but there are many problems relating to tissue rejection and the toxic drugs which are used to suppress rejection.

Local factors   Conditions such as:

1. *Uterine fibroids* which inhibit implantation of the ovum
2. *Cervical erosions* which affect the pH of secretions to the detriment of the sperm
3. *Congenital abnormalities* of the vagina, cervix or uterus which prevent the meeting of sperm or ovum.

The treatment here is that of the cause, with remedial surgery for congenital abnormalities where possible.

Despite modern diagnostic treatment, the cause of much infertility (approximately 10%) remains unknown and, despite modern scientific methods, much treatment remains unsuccessful. For many couples, infertility remains a problem with which they have to come to terms. For those who would like to adopt a child, the number of available babies are too few and it was to solve this problem that the programme of in vitro fertilisation was commenced.

Causes of male infertility

Spermatozoa are about 12 weeks old before they are ejaculated. The health of the male, 3 months before a pregnancy is planned, is therefore important. Possible causes of male infertility are listed below:

Defective spermatogenesis

Seminal fluid analysis may reveal:

1. *Sperm count below 20 million per millilitre* of seminal fluid
2. *Abnormal sperm count of more than 40%* – these are specific defects of head, mid-piece or tail. This may be due to germinal cell aplasia, 'sloughing' or a congenital defect, or some cause which cannot be defined
3. *Seminal fluid volume ejected is less than 2 ml*
4. *Chemical content of seminal fluid is unsatisfactory*, e.g. glucose, cholesterol or hyaluronidase levels are abnormal and the pH too high or low.

Postcoital tests may demonstrate:

1. *Less than 40% of sperm mobile 2 hours after intercourse.* This may be because they are unable to penetrate the cervical mucus
2. *No sperm still mobile 24 hours following intercourse.* There is frequently a temporary aspermatogenesis following an acute febrile illness.

Obstruction

1. *Congenital* occlusion of ducts or tubules
2. Occlusion of ducts or tubules caused by *acute or chronic inflammatory conditions* which affect the basement membrane or the muscular walls of the seminiferous tubules, e.g. orchitis, prostatic infection, gonococcal infection. This is one of the commonest causes of male infertility
3. *Other pathogenic conditions*, e.g. tumours, nutritional or vitamin deficiency diseases, radiation

Inability to achieve intercourse or ejaculation

1. Physical factors such as hypospadias, epispadias, deviation of the penis as in priapism or Peyronie's disease
2. Psychological factors causing inability to achieve or maintain an erection
3. Chronic alcoholism

Simple factors

Occasionally quite simple factors such as wearing tight-fitting jeans, taking baths which are too hot or a change of environment to a tropical climate may produce external conditions (heat) which are unfavourable for healthy sperm production.

ARTIFICIAL INSEMINATION AND IN VITRO FERTILISATION

The midwife is not likely to be involved with these techniques but an understanding of some of the terminology is required if any intelligent discussion is to take place during the course of her work and study. These are some of the more common terms used:

1. *AIH* (artificial insemination by the husband): The insertion into the uterus of sperm from the husband in a procedure other than sexual intercourse. The objective is to achieve pregnancy when intercourse is impossible.

2. *AID* (artificial insemination by a donor, a man other than the woman's husband): The objective is to achieve pregnancy when the husband is sterile or not able to achieve successful intercourse. The sperm are inserted by surgical means.

3. *Superovulation*: the production of several ova during one menstrual cycle by the use of such drugs as clomiphene or menotrophin,. This is in order to increase the possibility of pregnancy when fertilisation is initiated in vitro.

4. *IVF* (in vitro fertilisation): 'In vitro' means 'in glass'. Sperm and ovum are united in a test tube or glass dish under laboratory conditions for subsequent transfer to the woman's uterus.

5. *Freezing*: means the storage of sperm, ova and fertilised ova at very low temperatures. This is to reduce the need for repeated procedures in order to obtain them.

6. *Egg donation*: Mature ova are obtained from a donor, fertilised in vitro with sperm from the patient's husband and the embryo is then transferred to the uterus of his infertile wife.

7. *Embryo donation*: Both ova and sperm are donated and fertilised in vitro then subsequently transferred to the uterus of the woman who is to bear the child.

8. *Surrogate mother* (surrogate = deputy): A fertile woman carries and gives birth to a child and then surrenders it to the parents who have requested the arrangement. The child may or may not be the genetic child from the father and/or mother. Genetic parents can be quite different to the parents who want the child. Emotional, legal and moral problems can sometimes arise.

9. *Cloning*: The production of two or more genetically identical individuals. Ethical problems arise regarding sex-selection and the production of 'super' beings. In animals, 'cloning' is being used.

10. *Spare gametes or embryos*: 'Waste' products of infertility treatment! Ethical and legal considerations are still not resolved regarding their usage for medical and commercial research. Some are used for 'donation' to other infertile couples. The transplant of fetal tissue into patients with defined medical problems has already come under attack.

11. *Primitive streak*: The Warnock Report defines this as 'a heaping up of cells at one end of the embryonic disc on the 14th or

15th day after fertilisation'. They used this stage of development as the deciding factor in setting 14 days as the time when experimentation should stop.

12. *GIFT* (gamete intrafallopian transfer): Ova and sperm are mixed and inserted into the fallopian tube, where fertilisation takes place. There is then no creation of an embryo in laboratory conditions. It can only be used where the potency of the tubes is not a problem but is suitable for about 50% of those with fertility problems. Results are comparable to IVF, with implantation of three oocytes having the highest rate of success.

It is essential that couples who are selected for IVF programmes are able to accept ethically, emotionally and physically all that the procedure involves and they must be given a full explanation of frequent and wearying hospital visits which must of necessity be at uncertain times and dates. They must be intelligent enough to understand and co-operate with all the procedures that will be required and psychologically strong enough to forego feelings of guilt if ova are obtained but not fertilised successfully or if the embryo does not implant. Only about 25% of embryos implant successfully.

Culture of ova

1. Ova are obtained after 'superovulation' treatment, placed in culture fluid and left in an incubator for 5–12 hours to become 'mature'.

2. Spermatozoa are 'washed' so that the outer coat of the sperm head is cast off. They are then left in culture fluid for 1–2 hours.

3. About 50 000 sperm are placed with the ova and the cells are then returned to the incubator, where the sperm break down the zona pellucida and normal fertilisation should occur.

Development and implantation

48 hours after the ova have been fertilised, cleavage division will have produced a zygote containing eight cells and transfer to the uterus is commonly carried out at this stage. As many as five ova may be fertilised but usually no more than three are transferred.

REVISION QUESTIONS

Describe the structure and functions of the testes. What conditions might result in male sterility?

Make an illustrated comparison between the surgical procedures of male and female sterilisation.

Describe how the contraceptive 'pill' works. Name three other contraceptive methods.

Describe two treatments for female infertility.

At which time in the menstrual cycle is pregnancy

a) most likely to occur

b) least likely to occur?

Show how pregnancy may be prevented by the administration of a hormone.

Discuss the advantages and disadvantages of three different methods of contraception.

What factors may influence the choice of contraception for a woman and her partner following the birth of their first baby?

Discuss the role of the midwife in advising parents on family planning following the birth of their baby. (Should the midwife refer rather than advise?)

What similarities and what differences occur in the life cycles of the oocyte and spermatocyte.

Describe the methods of contraception which are available. What factors would you take into consideration when a postnatal woman asks for advice?

Write short notes on:

Counselling prior to sterilisation
Use of ultrasound to assess fertility
In vitro fertilisation.

REFERENCES AND FURTHER READING

Books and reports

Anon 1991 Regulations in the embryo bill. British Medical Journal 302: 1213

Billings E, Westmore A 1988 The Billings method of natural family planning: controlling fertility without drugs or devices. Thorsons, Wellingborough

Cowper A, Young C 1989 Family planning: fundamentals for health professionals. Chapman & Hall, London

Goldstein M, Feldberg M 1982 The vasectomy book: a complete guide to decision making. Turnstone Press, Wellingborough

Gray J 1990 A conflict in embryo (main issues of the Warnock report). Nursing Standard (Feb 28): 18–19

Guillebaud J 1986 Contraception: your questions answered. Churchill Livingstone, Edinburgh

Hayman S 1989 Vasectomy and sterilization: what you need to know. Thorsons, Wellingborough

Houghton D, Houghton P 1987 Coping with childlessness. Allen & Unwin, London

Kane P 1983 The Which? guide to birth control. Consumers' Association, London

Loudon N 1991 Handbook of family planning, 2nd edn. Churchill Livingstone, Edinburgh

Mealyea M 1987 A child – at any cost? Kingsway, Eastbourne

Snowden R, Snowden E 1984 The gift of a child. Allen & Unwin, London

Snowden R, Mitchell G D, Snowden E 1983 Artificial reproduction: a social investigation. Allen & Unwin, London

Warnock, M 1984 A question of life: the Warnock report on human fertilisation and embryology. Blackwell, Oxford

Articles

Aitken J 1988 Future developments in contraception. Practitioner 232: 46–52

Ah-Moye M, Craft I 1988 The GIFT technique – a new fertility option? Practitioner 232: 67–68; 71–72

Bashir Q 1988 Multi-cultural aspects of contraception. Update (1 Sept): 406–410

Benster R, Schmaroth A 1989 To use or not to use: a review of contraception as a psychological conflict. Maternal and Child Health (June): 62–64

Burley J K 1988 HIV positive women and contraception. British Journal of Family Planning 14(2): 50–54

Connor P 1991 Is IVF good medicine. Ethics and Medicine 27(2): 11–13

Dewart P J, London N B 1987 Contraception and lactation. Midwife, Health Visitor and Community Nurse (Aug): 334–337

Davis P 1991 Emergency contraception. British Medical Journal 302: 1082–1083

Duncan P 1987 Odd man out. Nursing Times (Jan 14): 39–40

Edelman R 1990 Emotional aspects of IVF procedures. Journal of Reproduction and Infertility Psychology (July/Sept): 161–173

Editorial 1987 Clinical status of IVF, GIFT and related techniques. Lancet ii: 946–947

Editorial 1990 The future of IVF and embryo research. Midwife, Health Visitor and Community Nurse (Sept): 364–366

Guillebaud J 1988 Present and future trends in contraception: the midwife's role in improving contraceptive efficiency. Professional Nurse (April): 222

Houston M et al 1980 The contraceptive effects of lactation. Nursing Times 76: 1231–1232

McLaughlin M 1989 Gamete intra-fallopian transfer. A treatment for infertility. Midwives' Chronicle 102: 23

McLaughlin M 1987 Gift of life: IVF, GIFT and intraperitoneal and intrauterine insemination for human infertility. IPPF Research in Reproduction (Jan) 1

Reynolds M 1988 Contraception: choices. Nursing (Jan): 948–951

Szarewski A 1989 Advances in contraception. Nursing Standard (13 May): 21–22

Szarewski A, Guillebaud J 1991 Contraception: current state of the art. British Medical Journal 302: 1224–1226

Updale A 1988 If the cap fits. Pediatrics (Nov): 133–135

Wolf F 1991 Contraceptive choices after childbirth. Parents (Feb): 80–84

Advice centres

British Association for Counselling, 37A Sheep Street, Rugby

British Pregnancy Advisory Service

Brook Advisory Centre

Family Planning Information Service

Health Education Council

John Wyeth Family Planning Service

LIFE, 35 Kenilworth Road, Leamington Spa

Margaret Pyke Centre for Study and Training in Family Planning, 27–35 Mortimer Street, London W1

Salvation Army Counselling Service, London (includes psychosexual counselling)

12 Early development of the placenta and chorion

(Plate 7A, B and C)

Spermatozoa Millions of spermatozoa, tadpole-like structures, are deposited by the male in the vagina during sexual intercourse. Each sperm is mature and carries 23 chromosomes in its nucleus.

The acidity of the vaginal fluid (pH 4.5) destroys many of the weaker or malformed sperm and many more may not reach the uterus because they cannot swim against the fluid currents. The strongest reach the fallopian tubes in a few hours and retain their fertilising ability for at least 72 hours, although some have been known to survive for 4 days. It has been demonstrated that the interstitial portion of the tube has a very favourable environment for the sperm and if they do not encounter an ovum before reaching that point, they cluster there. Fertilisation, however, takes place most commonly in the ampulla.

Ovum At ovulation the fimbriae of the fallopian tube approach the ovary and draw the ovum into the lumen. Once there it is carried towards the cavity of the uterus, partly by sweeping movements of the cilia and partly by the peristaltic action of the muscular tubular walls.

Fertilisation (Fig. 12.1) The spermatozoa that surround the ovum produce **hyaluronidase**, an enzyme that breaks down the protective protoplasm of the ovum in order to make penetration of the cell a little easier. It breaks down the corona radiata and facilitates penetration of the zona pellucida for one sperm only. As soon as contact between sperm head and ovum is established an antigen-type reaction takes place between the two cells so that they 'clump'. No other sperm is then able to penetrate the ovum.

The body and tail of the sperm separate from the head as soon as access to the ovum has been gained.

As soon as the two cells have united, the second polar spindle in the nucleus of the ovum undergoes its second meiotic division and is able to fuse with the nucleus of the sperm so that the diploid number of chromosomes is restored.

A further polar body (usually referred to as the second polar body) is formed as the result of the second meiotic division and its presence in the perivitelline space denotes that fertilisation has occurred. Like the first polar body, it normally degenerates. Both the fetus and the placenta, together with its appendages of amniotic

171

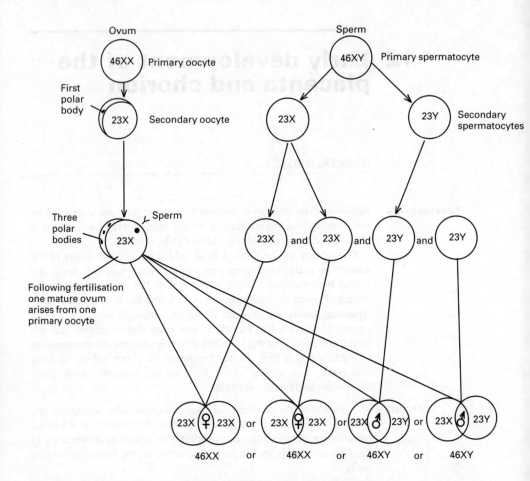

Fig. 12.1 Maturation of ovum and sperm, fertilisation and sex determination,

membrane, chorionic membrane, amniotic fluid and umbilical cord, are derived from this one fertilised cell.

EARLY DEVELOPMENT OF THE PLACENTA
(Fig. 12.2 A–H)

The zygote   The **zygote** is the name given to the fertilised ovum. Within a few hours, and still within the fallopian tube, it undergoes a series of cleavage divisions known as **mitosis**. In this type of cell division, the nucleus divides into two so that two new cells are formed, each with an identical set of chromosomes. This is the method by which all body cells except the **gametes** (ovum and sperm) are produced.

The morula   The **morula** is produced by continued reproduction of the zygote cell until it resembles a berry. Cell division is aided by progesterone from the corpus luteum which, together with oestrogen, is pre-

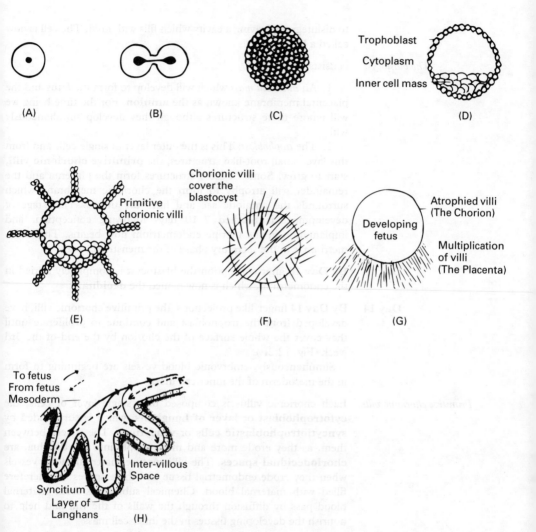

Fig. 12.2 Early stages of placental development: (A) penetration of ovum of sperm – zygote (B) cell division (C) morula (D) blastocyst (E) blastocyst with primitive chorionic villi (F) blastocyst ready to embed (G) primitive placenta and chorion (H) detailed structure of chorionic villus.

paring the uterine endometrium to receive a fertilised ovum. At the eight-cell stage the morula is about 2 mm in diameter and contains over 1000 different types of protein. It is still contained within the zona pellucida, rather like an egg within a shell, and is supported by its own cytoplasm which contains progesterone. 6–7 days after fertilisation the developing morula comes to lie adjacent to the endometrium which is in its secretory phase. It begins to embed by means of its own invasive properties which interact with the now 'sticky' surface of the uterine lining.

By the end of the first week, some inner cells in the morula begin to disintegrate, leaving a cavity which fills with fluid. The cell is now called a **blastocyst**.

The blastocyst consists of:

1. An *inner cell mass* which will develop to form the fetus and the placental membrane known as the **amnion**. For the time being we will ignore these structures although they develop simultaneously with

2. The *trophoblast*: This is the outer layer of single cells and from this layer small root-like structures, the **primitive chorionic villi**, start to grow. Some of these structures form the placenta and the remainder will atrophy to form the chorionic membrane which surrounds the amniotic sac and lines the uterus. This stage of development is reached 7–10 days following conception, and implantation in the uterine endometrium now begins. The endometrium is in the secretory phase of the menstrual cycle.

Day 10 **By Day 10** after conception the blastocyst is completely buried in the endometrium, which is now named the **decidua**.

Day 14 **By Day 14** finger-like projections, the primitive chorionic villi, have developed from the trophoblast and continue to proliferate until they cover the whole surface of the chorion by the end of the 3rd week (Fig. 12.2F).

Simultaneously, embryonic blood vessels are beginning to form in the mesoderm of the inner cell mass.

Primitive chorionic villi Each chorionic villus is composed of a single layer of cells, the **cytotrophoblast** or **layer of Langhans**, which is surrounded by **syncytiotrophoblastic cells** or **syncytium**. The spaces between them, as they erode more and more deeply into the decidua, are **choriodecidual spaces**. The villi rupture maternal blood vessels when they erode endometrial tissue and these spaces are therefore filled with maternal blood. Chemical substances from maternal blood pass by diffusion through the walls of the villi and help to nourish the developing tissues in the inner cell mass.

3rd week **During the 3rd week** branching of the primitive chorionic villi occurs. These branches are called **secondary primitive chorionic villi** and blood vessels begin to form within them.

Tertiary chorionic villi are so called when the blood vessels have formed and these blood vessels become connected to the embryonic blood vessels in the body stalk. (The vessels in the stalk develop to form **two arteries** and **one umbilical vein** for the fetus.)

Some chorionic villi continue to bury more deeply into the decidua and are known as **anchoring villi**. They have no blood vessels within them since their task is just to stabilise the developing placenta. Other villi branch from them, the spaces between them being called **intervillous spaces**.

In the **uterus** the pregnant endometrium, renamed the decidua, is now differentiated into three areas:

1. *Decidua basalis* lies below the area where the chorionic villi first embedded
2. *Decidua capsularis* lies above the embryonic sac
3. *Decidua vera* (or *parietalis*) lines the remainder of the uterine cavity.

8th week

Until the 8th week of pregnancy, chorionic villi surround the whole of the embryonic sac. Then further changes occur.

Chorion laeve

As the inner cell mass continues to increase in size, the decidua capsularis is pushed continually outwards into the uterine cavity until it lies adjacent to the decidua vera. As the chorion laeve lies on the inner surface of the decidua capsularis, it too lines the uterine cavity and develops to form the placental membrane known as the **chorion**.

Chorion frondosum

In the decidua basalis, where a rich blood supply is maintained, these villi continue to multiply and develop rapidly. Those that bed deeply in the decidua basalis become firmly anchored by the 12th week of pregnancy, so **stabilising** the developing placenta. Others branch outwards allowing maternal blood to circulate freely between them to provide **nourishment** for further growth of placenta and fetus.

14th week

By the 14th week of pregnancy the structure of the placenta is fully developed and it occupies about one-third of the uterine wall. From the end of the 8th week of pregnancy the primitive placenta has been secreting oestrogen, progesterone and relaxin.

Chorionic gonadotrophin

From the **9th week**, as the chorionic villi embed in the uterine wall, a hormone called **chorionic gonadotrophin** (hCG) is produced. Its function is to stimulate growth and hormone secretion of the corpus luteum and so maintain the pregnancy until the placenta is fully functioning.

Chorionic gonadotrophin is secreted in increasing amounts until the end of the first trimester of pregnancy, after which it declines. Because it is produced only by the trophoblast and is excreted in the urine, its presence on urinalysis is a positive indication of pregnancy and this fact is used as the basis for immunological pregnancy tests.

16th week

From the 16th week onwards the number and size of the fetal blood vessels increase while the walls of the villi become thinner so that, during the mid-trimester, the 'permeability' of the placenta is, in fact, increased. During the last 4 weeks of pregnancy, however, it is reduced again as fibrin deposits are laid down in its tissues.

20th week

After the 20th week the placenta continues to increase in circumference rather than to thicken, until at full term it is about 23 cm in diameter, a round, flat organ about 2 cm thick in the centre but thinner at the circumference.

Two points of interest might be made here:

1. The erosion of the maternal blood vessels by the chorionic villi results in the presence of free blood in the tissues. Yet this

does not cause the formation of a haematoma or any other problems.

2. The walls of the chorionic villi are very often referred to as the placental barrier. **The placenta is not a barrier**; it acts as a **permeable membrane**.

PATHOLOGICAL DEVELOPMENT OF THE PLACENTA

Hydatidiform mole

During the first few weeks of placental development there is a proliferative growth of the chorionic villi and each tiny, root-like structure terminates in a sac of fluid. Because of the rapid growth of the trophoblastic layer, the inner cell mass is absorbed and the fetus does not develop. The mole increases in size much more rapidly than the fetus would develop and the size of the uterus is therefore much greater than the period of amenorrhoea suggests, but no fetal parts can be felt. Due to proliferation of the chorionic villi, the amount of chorionic gonadotrophin is greatly increased and a pregnancy diagnosis test will be positive even at 1–1000 dilution.

Diagnosis is made on the result of this test following the occurrence of vaginal bleeding, also taking into consideration the patient's history, which includes a feeling of general ill-health and excessive morning sickness. It is confirmed by ultrasound or chorionic villi biopsy with histological examination of tissue. Pre-eclampsia often develops as early as the 16th week of pregnancy. In approximately 10% of patients there is a risk of malignancy (**chorionepithelioma**).

If spontaneous abortion does not occur, the patient is admitted to hospital and the uterus is evacuated by vacuum extraction if the condition has been diagnosed before 12 weeks. After this time, labour is induced with an intravenous drip using prostaglandin E_2. Preparation for intrapartum or postpartum haemorrhage must be made, i.e. blood must be cross-matched and readily available for use.

Urine and serum tests are then carried out over the next 2 years to estimate the hCG levels. During this time the patient is advised not to become pregnant. The hCG levels should remain low. Should the levels in urine or blood samples rise, hysterectomy is carried out if the patient is certain that she wants no more children. Alternatively, treatment by chemotherapy is indicated and has proved successful. Drugs are continued until 2 months after the hCG levels have returned to normal.

REVISION QUESTIONS

Refer to Chapters 9, 10, 13, 14.

REFERENCES AND FURTHER READING

Books and reports

Netter F H 1965 CIBA collection of medical illustrations. CIBA Foundation, New York

Williams P L, Wendall Smith C P, Treadgold S 1984 Basic human embryology. Pitman Medical, London

See also Chapter 14

Articles

Atrasm M et al 1986 Epidemiology of hydatidiform mole during early gestation. American Journal of Obstetrics and Gynecology 154: 906–909

Bracken M B 1987 Incidence and aetiology of hydatidiform mole: an epidemiological review. British Journal of Obstetrics and Gynaecology 94(12): 1123–1135

Enders A 1986 Cytology of human implantation. IPPF Research in Reproduction (Sept)

Parazzini F et al 1986 Parental age and risk of partial and complete hydatidiform mole. British Journal of Obstetrics and Gynaecology 93: 582–585

13 The placenta at term

(Plate 8)

Situation
Before delivery the placenta is normally situated in the upper uterine segment. Its position can be confirmed when ultrasound examination is carried out as a routine measure in pregnancy. A repeat scan is made in the last trimester if the first examination shows the placenta to be encroaching into the lower segment. In many instances it is then found to be totally contained within the upper uterine segment.

Shape
It is a flat, roughly circular structure.

Size
The placenta is approximately 22 cm in diameter. It is about 2 cm thick in the centre but gets thinner towards the circumference. It weighs about 0.5 kg.

Structure

Maternal surface
(Fig. 13.1A)
In utero the maternal surface of the placenta lies next to the uterus, deeply embedded in the decidua. On inspection, following delivery, the chorionic villi (which have already been described in detail on p. 174 ff.) are arranged in lobes, or **cotyledons**. The grooves separating the cotyledons are called **sulci**. This surface is dark red in colour, due to maternal blood in the spaces between the villi and to fetal blood in the vessels within each villus. The intervillous spaces contain approximately 150 ml of blood which is changed at least three times per minute. At full term this surface feels rather rough to the touch because, having reached its full development by the 28th week of pregnancy, it then begins slowly to degenerate. Fibrin is deposited over the villi and deposits of calcium can be seen with the naked eye at term. If a large area of placental tissue is affected and becomes fibrosed and white, it is called an **infarct**. The area becomes inefficient and ceases to function.

Fetal surface (Fig. 13.1B)
This faces the baby in utero and is distinguished on inspection after delivery by its bluish-grey colour and its smooth, shiny surface. The umbilical cord is inserted into this surface, usually in the centre, and blood vessels can be seen radiating from the cord to be lost deep in the substance of the placenta before reaching its circumference. The amniotic membrane covers the fetal surface and can be stripped back from the chorion as far as the insertion of the umbilical cord. The chorion, being derived from the same tropho-

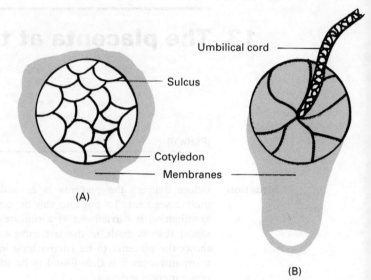

Fig. 13.1 Placenta at term
(A) maternal surface (B) fetal
surface.

blastic layer as the placenta, is continuous with the placental edge and cannot be separated from it.

The amnion   is a tough transparent membrane, very difficult to tear. It lines the amniotic cavity, covers the placenta and umbilical cord and secretes the amniotic fluid. Its derivation is described on pages 174 and 208.

The chorion   is an opaque, thin, friable membrane, although it does appear to be thicker than the amnion. Because it is so easily torn, small pieces are sometimes detached during delivery and retained in utero. Its derivation is described on page 175.

Functions

Exchange system   1. *Nutrients*: The placenta has many enzymes and is able to synthesise:
- *Carbohydrates*: glucose passes across the placental membrane very easily but more complex carbohydrates need to be broken down. Some is stored as glycogen for fetal needs
- *Proteins* are broken down into amino acids that the fetus can use
- *Fats* are more difficult to simplify and, with *fat-soluble vitamins,* pass to the fetus only slowly
- *Water-soluble vitamins* B and C are easily transmitted to the fetus, as are
- *Mineral salts.*
2. *Waste products* are returned to the maternal circulation via the chorionic villi:
- The nitrogenous products of nutrients
- Bilirubin, the product of broken-down red blood cells.

3. *Gases*: Maternal oxyhaemoglobin is broken down into its components, oxygen and haemoglobin.

- *Oxygen* is diffused across the placental barrier to form fetal oxyhaemoglobin. 20–35 ml of oxygen per minute is passed to the fetus, the actual amount being dependent upon the condition of maternal blood vessels and the structures involved in placental interchange. Smoking, for instance, is known to reduce the amount of oxygen which a mother transmits to her fetus
- *Carbon dioxide* is returned to the placenta for excretion into the maternal circulation.

'Supplies' to the fetus are carried in the umbilical vein. Waste products are returned via the umbilical arteries.

Protective system

Protects fetal tissues from maternal rejection The fetal tissues, with their different genetic structure, would be regarded as 'foreign' and rejected by the mother were it not for the protection supplied by the placenta. A good deal of research has centred on this fact.

It has been demonstrated in the laboratory that the activity of lymphocytes can be suppressed by hormones such as oestrogens, progesterone, prolactin and hCG. It does seem, therefore, that the placental hormones combat any likelihood of the rejection of fetal tissue.

Partial protection from infection The placenta transmits maternal antibodies which will give the fetus a passive immunity to those diseases for which the mother herself has acquired an immunity. This protection is carried into the early months of life. However, the fetus is not protected from **viruses** such as rubella and varicella or from the **spirochaete** of syphilis. In the event of rubella virus being transmitted in the early developmental period of the fetus, there are likely to be defects affecting the heart, eyes and ears. If syphilis is transmitted and untreated, the infant will be syphilitic, a rare condition in the UK, but not totally unknown. If she has already been sensitised, a rhesus-negative mother will produce **antibodies** in her circulatory system to the rhesus antigen if the fetus is rhesus-positive. The placenta is unable to bar the antibodies and so, diffusing into the fetal system, they destroy red cells, causing varying degrees of anaemia from the very mild condition to **hydrops fetalis** if the condition is undiagnosed or untreated. Here again, this is very unlikely in the UK but can arise in areas of the world where mothers are not seen until they are in labour.

The causative organisms of syphilis and tuberculosis and rhesus antibodies all affect the function of the placenta and make it abnormal in appearance.

Secretory system

Human chorionic gonadotrophin (hcG) Produced as early as the ninth day following conception, this hormone reaches its peak on day 60. Levels then fall and remain low until the end of pregnancy. Its function is to maintain the corpus luteum until the placenta can take over its production of oestrogen and progesterone. As mentioned earlier, hCG is excreted in the urine and forms the basis of immunological pregnancy diagnosis tests.

Oestrogen Levels of this hormone rise throughout pregnancy and help to effect endometrial changes in the early weeks. Oestrogen also develops the secretory function of the breasts. Late in pregnancy the raised maternal oestrogens are dominant and, with fetal steroids, stimulate prostaglandin production. This in turn stimulates the production of oxytocin from the posterior pituitary gland. Oestrogens also increase the sensitivity of uterine muscle to oxytocin which initiates uterine contractions and the onset of labour.

Progesterone Large amounts of progesterone are synthesised from maternal cholesterol but the placenta lacks the enzymes which are necessary to convert some of it into oestrogens (oestriol, oestrone and oestradiol). The synthesis is actually carried out by the immature fetal adrenal glands. It seems strange that although the fetus cannot manufacture his own oestrogen he can convert and use his mother's!

As well as aiding fetal development these hormones act on uterine muscle and develop breast tissue. The main function of progesterone is to act on tissues which have already been receptive to oestrogen.

Relaxin Relaxin is a hormone very similar in construction to insulin, and until recently it has been difficult to isolate one from the other. Relaxin is produced by the theca and luteinised granulosa cells of the corpus luteum and its production is continued throughout pregnancy. It has a general effect in the preparation of the genital tract for pregnancy and labour, softening and relaxing connective tissue. It rises to a peak before the onset of labour and helps to effect ripening and effacement of the cervix as well as rupturing of the membranes.

Human placental lactogen (hPL) As the placental production of hCG falls, so its production of hPL is increased. Levels of the hormone then continue to rise throughout pregnancy until the 36th week, then fall again.

This hormone is associated with changes in the maternal metabolism of glucose, which are of advantage to the mother, and is also associated with growth hormone.

Stabilisation Those chorionic villi which pass deeply into the decidua and anchor the placenta firmly (see Ch. 12, p. 174) stabilise the structure which is so vital for fetal development.

ABNORMALITIES OF PLACENTAL DEVELOPMENT

Placenta succenturiata
(Fig. 13.2A)

This is a placenta in which an accessory cotyledon develops away from the main placental structure. Blood vessels travel across the

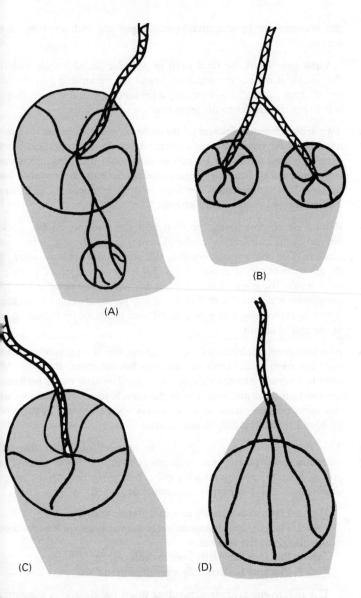

ig. 13.2 Abnormalities of placental development (A) placenta
uccenturiata (B) placenta bipartita (C) placenta circumvallata (D) placenta
elamentosa.

membranes connecting the succenturiate lobe with the main placenta. Two complications occur with this abnormality:

1. *The accessory lobe might be retained in utero* when the placenta is
expelled, giving rise to postpartum haemorrhage and/or uterine infection and secondary postpartum haemorrhage.

2. *Fetal anoxia can be caused* either by the presenting part of
the fetus pushing against the vessels connecting the lobe with

the placenta, or by the membranes rupturing and involving the vessels.

Vasa praevia is the term used to describe blood vessels within the placental membrane which lie below the presenting part. If the membranes rupture, involving these presenting blood vessels, there is consequent danger to the fetus because of blood loss.

Placenta bipartita
(Fig. 13.2B)

Two separate areas of placental tissue develop but there are no connecting blood vessels between them. There is one umbilical cord which divides, sending a branch to each lobe, thus distinguishing this abnormality from twin placentae where two cords would be present. No complications are likely to arise with this abnormality; it is mentioned purely out of interest.

Placenta circumvallata
(Fig. 13.2C)

During development, the amnion and the chorion double back around the circumference of the placenta, giving the appearance of a collar. The chorion is, therefore, still continuous with the edge of the placenta but its attachment is folded back on to the fetal surface. As a result, the edge of the placenta is more easily detached from the uterine wall and this may result in antepartum haemorrhage, the actual causation not being recognised until the placenta is examined at the end of labour.

Placenta velamentosa
(Figs 13.2D and 13.5D)

Also known as velamentous cord insertion, this is an abnormality of cord insertion rather than of placental development. Because the cord is inserted into the membranes, blood vessels travel between the cord and the placenta across the membranes. The dangers of this condition are those of vasa praevia – pressure on, or rupture of, blood vessels, leading to fetal anoxia.

Placenta praevia
(Fig. 13.3A, B, C, D)

This is an abnormality of developmental position rather than of placental development, and is therefore mentioned only briefly. It occurs when the placenta is lying either partly or wholly in the lower uterine segment. Four types are usually described.

Type 1: Placenta lies partly in lower uterine segment
Type 2: Placenta lies mostly in lower uterine segment and reaches to the margin of the internal os
Type 3: Placenta lies partly over the internal os
Type 4: Placenta lies centrally over the internal os.

The risk to the fetus is dependent upon the degree of placental separation and consequent blood loss as the uterus contracts. Clearly, with types 3 and 4, elective caesarean section is always the chosen method of delivery.

PATHOLOGICAL CONDITIONS OF THE PLACENTA

Premature degeneration

Maternal diseases such as essential hypertension and renal disease cause a narrowing of the lumen of blood vessels and the blood

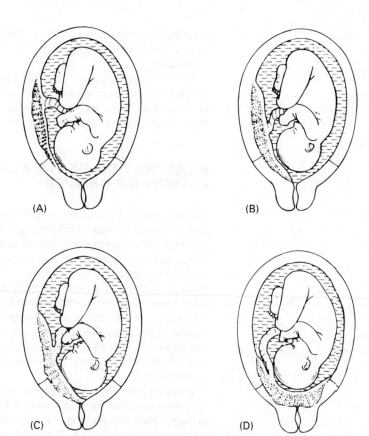

(A) (B)

(C) (D)

Fig. 13.3 Placenta praevia: (A) Type 1 – placenta lies partly in lower uterine segment (B) Type 2 – placenta mostly in lower uterine segment; reaches to margin of internal os (C) Type 3 – placenta lies partly over internal os (D) Type 4 – placenta lies centrally over internal os.

supply to the placenta is therefore diminished. Inadequate placental development occurs and large areas of tissue may die, leading to fetal death and the termination of pregnancy before the 28th week.

Infarcts It has already been stated that the placenta begins to degenerate at the 28th week of pregnancy. More extensive degeneration occurs in association with pre-eclampsia because the disease causes arteriole spasm and large infarcted areas result in placental inefficiency. Labour is usually induced before term because the fetus fails to grow in utero, and further degeneration of the placenta might result in fetal death before or during labour.

When pregnancy is prolonged for more than 40 weeks, extensive calcareous degeneration occurs of the postmature placenta and this too can cause fetal anoxia before or during labour.

Oedema A large, pale, waterlogged placenta is always associated with severe haemolytic disease of the newborn. Its weight may be equal to half that of the fetus. The term used to describe the oedematous fetus is **hydrops fetalis**.

Excessive size 1. A large placenta is found in association with *syphilis* when it is also described as being pale and greasy- looking. On microscopic examination spirochaetes will be found and the chorionic villi have a characteristic appearance which is readily recognised by a technician.

2. It is sometimes said that the placenta of a *diabetic mother* is larger than the normal, but this is not always true. When found in association with the large fetus of the diabetic mother it is most probably due to the growth factor of the pituitary gland.

EXAMINATION OF THE PLACENTA FOLLOWING DELIVERY

Labour cannot be said to be complete until the placenta and membranes have been carefully inspected and checked following delivery. If there is any doubt that small pieces of placental tissue or membrane have been retained in the uterus, the placenta must be retained for inspection by the medical officer. All placentae showing abnormal pathology should also be retained for inspection. These facts must be recorded on the mother's notes. Placental tissue retained in the uterus is likely to give rise to postpartum haemorrhage since the uterus cannot contract and retract effectively. Expulsion of retained products may be aided by the administration of an oxytocic drug or by evacuation of the uterus under anaesthetic.

Retained pieces of membrane are usually expelled spontaneously. The mother should be told to watch for them when she uses the lavatory. Retained products of conception, if not expelled within 48 hours, give rise to infection and secondary postpartum haemorrhage.

THE UMBILICAL CORD

The umbilical cord is derived from the duct which forms between the amniotic sac and the yolk sac.

Situation The umbilical cord extends from the fetal surface of the placenta to the umbilical area of the fetus and is continuous with the fetal skin at that junction. It is normally inserted into the centre of the placenta.

Size At full term it measures 40–50 cm in length and is 1–2 cm in diameter.

Shape As its name implies, it is like a cord and has about 40 spiral twists in it.

Structure (Fig. 13.4)

Amnion covers the cord and is a continuation of that covering the fetal surface of the placenta. At the fetal end it is continuous with the skin

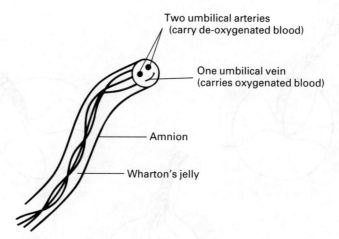

Two umbilical arteries
(carry de-oxygenated blood)

One umbilical vein
(carries oxygenated blood)

Amnion

Wharton's jelly

Fig. 13.4 Structure of the umbilical cord.

which covers the abdomen. Both skin and amniotic membrane derive from ectoderm.

Three blood vessels coil around each other within the cord and are continuous with the tiny vessels in the chorionic villi of the placenta. One umbilical vein transports oxygen and nutrients to the fetal circulatory system from maternal blood which lies in the choriodecidual spaces. Two umbilical arteries return waste products from the fetus to the placenta where they are assimilated into the maternal circulation for excretion.

Wharton's jelly surrounds the blood vessels. It is a jelly-like substance which, like the blood vessels, is derived from mesoderm. Wharton's jelly sometimes collects in small clusters and forms a false knot in the cord. It is the amount of jelly which makes the cord thick or thin.

Nerves and lymphatic vessels There are none in the cord.

Abnormalities of cord insertion (Fig. 13.5) Although the cord most frequently has a central insertion into the fetal surface of the placenta, it is sometimes inserted **laterally**. Less frequently it is inserted into the placental edge as a **battledore** insertion. More rarely still it is inserted into the membranes as a **velamentous** insertion or **placenta velamentosa** (Fig. 13.2D).

CARE OF THE CORD AFTER DELIVERY

When the infant is ready to be separated from the mother, two pairs of Spencer Wells artery forceps are applied to the cord and the cord is cut between them. Pulsations of the cord will cease because the external temperature causes contraction of the Wharton's jelly and blood vessels. The forceps on the maternal end of the cord prevent the mess which would be made if placental blood were to leak everywhere.

The forceps on the infant's end of the cord are to prevent blood

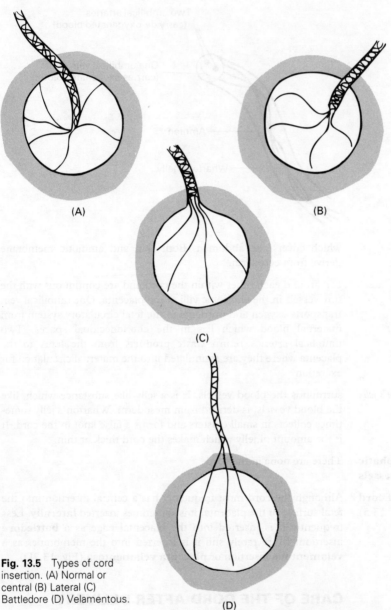

Fig. 13.5 Types of cord insertion. (A) Normal or central (B) Lateral (C) Battledore (D) Velamentous.

loss from his own circulation. An umbilical clamp or firm ligature is then applied to his end of the cord before the forceps are removed.

It is essential to maintain regular observations of the cord to ensure that there is no blood loss during the early postnatal hours.

The cord must always be examined by the midwife when she makes an examination of the placenta following delivery. The absence of a blood vessel in the cord is associated with fetal abnormalities.

REVISION QUESTIONS

Describe the functions of the placenta. How may the efficiency of the placenta be impaired?

Describe the appearance of the normal placenta at term. What anatomical and pathological changes may be seen in the placenta?

Describe the placenta at term. Enumerate its functions.

Describe the umbilical cord. What should a midwife do if the cord prolapses?

Describe a twin placenta at term. Why are the placenta and membranes so carefully examined after delivery?

Describe the structure of the umbilical cord. What complications involving the cord may be dangerous to the baby?

Describe the placenta. What abnormalities may occur? What is their significance?

What are the functions of the placenta? How may placental function be monitored in pregnancy?

Describe the anatomy and physiology of the placenta. What are its functions? Discuss how placental functions may be monitored in pregnancy. Describe the management and care of a woman whose uterine size is smaller than expected for the estimated gestational age.

Describe the placenta and membranes at term. Describe the functions of the mature placenta. How may placental function be assessed during pregnancy?

Write short notes on:

Succenturiate placenta
Functions of the placenta
Human chorionic gonadotrophin
Oestriol in pregnancy
Examination of the placenta and membranes
Placental function.

REFERENCES AND FURTHER READING

Articles

Al-Ghazali W et al 1988 Doppler assessment of the cardiac and uteroplacental circulations in normal and complicated pregnancies. British Journal of Obstetrics and Gynaecology 95(6): 575–580

Barr J 1984 The umbilical cord: to treat or not to treat. Midwives' Chronicle 97: 224–226

Botha M 1968 Management of the umbilical cord in labour. South African Journal of Obstetrics and Gynaecology (24 Aug): 30

Rivera-Alsina M E, Saldana L R, Maklad N, Korp S 1983 The use of ultrasound in the expectant management of abruptio placentae. American Journal of Obstetrics and Gynecology 146(8): 924–927

14 Development of the fetus, amniotic membrane and amniotic fluid

(Plate 7C)

DEVELOPMENT OF THE FETUS

Fertilisation The fertilisation of the ovum by the sperm has already been described in Chapter 12 but it is studied now in relation to fetal development.

Gestation period The human embryo requires approximately 280 days to reach maturity. To assess the **expected date of delivery** (EDD), when the woman has a regular 28-day menstrual cycle:

1. Take the **first** day of the last menstrual cycle (LMP) as 1 January
2. then **add** 7 days = 8 January
3. Count forward 9 months, commencing with the following month (i.e. February)
4. making EDD = 8 October.

If the menstrual cycle is shorter than 28 days, e.g. 24 days, subtract 4 days: i.e. EDD = 4 October

If the menstrual cycle is longer than 28 days, e.g. 30 days, add 2 days: i.e. EDD = 10 October

If the cycle is irregular, or the woman does not know when her last period was, it is impossible to calculate the EDD by this means.

Conception 23 chromosomes in the nucleus of the sperm unite with the 23 in the nucleus of the ovum at the moment of fertilisation. This restores the human somatic pattern of 46 chromosomes arranged in 23 pairs.

Chromosomes These consist of protein material and the genetic material commonly called DNA (deoxyribonucleic acid).

All chromosomes except those involved in sex determination are called **autosomes**. The chromosomes carry the **genes**.

Genes These are the microscopic particles of protoplasm contained within the chromosomes. They are arranged in pairs which may be **homozygous** or **heterozygous**. Because each chromosome carries hereditary material in its genes, not only the sex but the appearance and characteristics of the new child are determined at the very moment of conception and are conveyed from both parents.

191

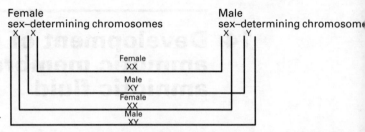

Fig. 14.1 Sex determination.

Sex determination
(Fig. 14.1)

This is the function of the sex chromosomes. One pair of chromosomes is sex-determining, those of the female being designated XX and those of the male XY. The sex will therefore be dependent upon the way in which the chromosomes split during meiosis and then combine again at fertilisation (p. 172). X from the female gamete (the ovum) pairing with X from the sperm will result in XX, a female child, while X from the female pairing with the Y from the sperm will result in XY, a male child. As the male carries the Y chromosome, it can be seen that it is the male partner who determines the sex of the children.

EARLY EMBRYONIC DEVELOPMENT
(Fig. 14.2A, B, C, D)

In the inner cell mass, 6–7 days after fertilisation, the **blastocyst** begins to embed in the uterus and is completely buried by the 10th day.

By this time there has been a differentiation of the cells composing the inner cell mass. The first stage in fetal development is the formation of two enclosed cavities which lie adjacent to each other, the amniotic sac and the yolk sac (Fig. 14.2A).

Ectoderm

lines the **amniotic sac**. It is a single layer of cells which is responsible for the growth of fetal skin, hair, nails, teeth, nerve tissue, including that of the sense organs, salivary glands, nasal cavity, lower part of the anal canal, the genital tract and the mammary glands.

Endoderm

lines the yolk sac and develops to form the digestive tract, liver, pancreas, larynx, trachea, lungs, bladder and urethra.

Mesoderm

This is the remainder of the tissue of the inner cell mass. Some of it lies around the embryonic plate. The further development of the mesoderm produces the circulatory and lymphatic systems, the skeleton, muscles, kidneys, ureters, sex organs and subcutaneous tissues of the skin. By an action similar to that of the single-celled amoeba ingesting food, the amniotic cavity alters its shape in order to surround the yolk sac and mesoderm and draw these tissues into itself.

Embryonic plate
(Fig. 14.2A)

Because the amniotic and yolk sacs are adjacent, some ectoderm of the amniotic cavity lies in contact with some of the endoderm of the

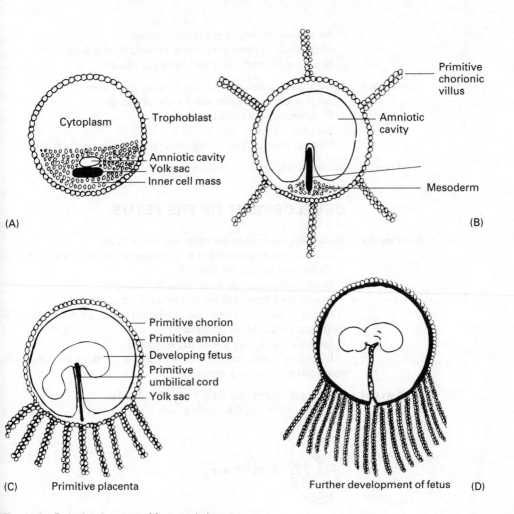

Fig. 14.2 Early development of fetus and placenta.

yolk sac. This area is known as the embryonic plate and is the site of fetal development.

FURTHER DEVELOPMENT OF THE EMBRYO

First 14 days   The blastocyst is nourished by its own cytoplasm.

Primitive blood vessels for the embryo begin to develop in the mesoderm.

14–28 days   Embryonic blood vessels connect up with blood vessels in the chorionic villi of the primitive placenta.

Embryo/maternal circulation is thus established and blood is circulating.

Head of embryo can be distinguished from the body.

Leg buds and then arm buds appear.

An attitude of flexion gradually appears.

Major body systems are present in rudimentary form.

Heart bulges from body and begins to pulsate.

28–42 days Length is approximately 12 mm by end of 6th week.

Arms begin to elongate and hands take shape.

Rudimentary eyes and ears appear.

Ears are apparent but set low.

First movements can be detected on ultrasound from 6 weeks.

8 weeks marks the end of the embryonic period.

DEVELOPMENT OF THE FETUS

8–10 weeks *Head* is approximately the same size as the body.

Neck is longer, so that chin is no longer in contact with the body.

Fingers and toes can be defined.

Ossification centres are developing in cartilage.

Eyelids are formed but are closed until the 25th week.

Intestines herniate into the umbilical cord because there is inadequate room in the abdomen.

Cord insertion is very low in the abdomen.

If mother's abdomen is palpated too forcefully, the fetus will **move away** (observed on scan).

12 weeks *Body length* is approximately 9 cm. *Weight* 14 g.

Fetal circulation is functioning fully.

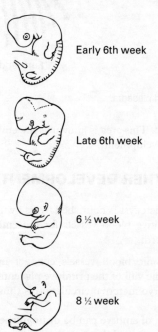

Early 6th week

Late 6th week

6 ½ week

8 ½ week

Fig. 14.3 Fetal development.

Renal tract begins to function.

Sucking and *swallowing* reflexes are present.

External genitalia are apparent and sex can be determined.

12–16 weeks *Body length* is approximately 16 cm by the 16th week. *Weight* 100 g.

Skin is so transparent that blood vessels can be seen through it.

Deposits of *subcutaneous fat* are laid down towards the 16th week.

Hair begins to appear on the head and lanugo on the body.

Legs are longer than the arms.

16–20 weeks *Rate of growth* begins to slow down.

Head is now erect and half the length of the trunk.

Facial features are distinctive with ears sited in normal position.

Eyelids, *eyebrows* and *finger nails* are all well developed.

Legs are in relative proportion with the body.

Skeleton is visible on X-ray examination (although X-ray is not used for diagnostic purposes).

Sebaceous glands are active and **vernix caseosa** covers the body.

Fetal movements are felt by the mother after the 18th week.

Fetal heart can be heard with the aid of a stethoscope after the 20th week.

Renal tract is functioning, 7–17 ml of urine being passed in 24 hours.

20–24 weeks *Skin* is very wrinkled because there is so little subcutaneous fat.

Lanugo becomes darker and vernix caseosa increases.

From 24 weeks onwards the fetus will *kick* in response to stimulation such as loud external noise.

He appears *soothed* if his mother listens to quiet tranquil music.

All *organs* are well developed.

Add saccharin to amniotic fluid and the fetus's swallowing rate doubles. Add lipidol and he grimaces!

24–28 weeks *Eyes* are open. *Eyebrows* and *lashes* well developed.

Hair covers his head.

More deposits of subcutaneous fat result in less wrinkling of skin.

The testes are descending from the abdomen into the scrotum at 28 weeks. A fetus born towards the end of this period still has quite a high mortality rate because of respiratory problems.

28–32 weeks *Lanugo* begins to diminish.

The body is beginning to become *more rounded* as fat is laid down.

Testes continue to descend.

32–36 weeks *Lanugo* has mostly been shed but the skin is still covered with vernix.

Testes of the male are in the scrotum by the 36th week.

The *ovaries* of the female are still above the pelvic brim.

Finger and *toe nails* reach the tip of the digits.

Umbilicus now lies more centrally in the abdomen.

36–40 weeks Ossification of skull bones is still not complete but this is an advantage and facilitates the passage of the fetus through the birth canal.

Fetal respiratory movements can be identified on ultrasound scanning. There are now adequate amounts of subcutaneous fat and the fetus gains almost a kilo during these weeks.

At birth   Many of the fetus's systems are still immature but:

- he is capable of free movement
- he can breathe and has a lusty cry
- he is anxious to feed at the breast
- within moments of birth he passes urine and meconium
- he responds to the stimulus of sight, sound and touch.

In appearance:

- he is plump and pink
- he has a little lanugo and a little vernix
- head, chest and abdomen are approximately each 35 cm in circumference
- his length is 50 cm
- his weight is approximately 3.5 kg.

WEIGHT AND LENGTH OF DEVELOPING FETUS (Table 14.1)

Length of the fetus   A helpful rule to provide a guide to relating the length of the fetus to the weeks of gestation is this. Between 12 and 20 weeks take the age in months, square it and that gives the approximate length in centimetres – crown to heels:

e.g. 12 weeks = 3 months 3^2 = 9 cm
16 weeks = 4 months 4^2 = 16 cm
20 weeks = 5 months 5^2 = 25 cm

After 20 weeks determine the age in months and multiply by 5:

24 weeks = 6 months × 5 = 30 cm
28 weeks = 7 months × 5 = 35 cm
32 weeks = 8 months × 5 = 40 cm
36 weeks = 9 months × 5 = 45 cm
40 weeks = 10 months × 5 = 50 cm

Table 14.1 Growth of fetus

Weeks	Length	Weight
12	9 cm	14 g
16	16 cm	100 g
20	25 cm	225 g
24	30 cm	680 g
28	35 cm	1.15 kg
32	40 cm	1.60 kg
36	45 cm	2.25 kg
40	50 cm	3.50 kg

Ultrasound can of course measure the length with accuracy.

Weight of the fetus See Table 14.1

ORIGINS OF CONSCIOUSNESS

During this decade a good deal of work has been carried out into the origins of consciousness and the shaping of personality during intrauterine life. Mother/baby bonding relationships were discussed briefly in relation to feeding experiences (Ch. 2, p. 13) but evidence does now show that bonding after birth is just the continuation of that begun during fetal life. In the fifth century BC Hippocrates stressed the importance to the pregnant woman and her fetus of listening to beautiful music and thinking beautiful thoughts. Leonardo da Vinci also had a good deal to say about antenatal influences on the fetus.

Relevant reading material is suggested in the reference section relating to this chapter.

MULTIPLE PREGNANCY

The incidence of twins in the UK is 1 in 80 pregnancies, although in some instances one twin may be aborted early in pregnancy while the other goes to full term.

While the term 'multiple pregnancy' is commonly taken to mean twin pregnancy, there have recently been instances of as many as eight live babies being delivered at the end of pregnancy. There is no doubt that the incidence of multiple pregnancy has increased since the use of drugs to stimulate ovulation in infertile women.

A twin pregnancy may result from the fertilisation either of a single ovum or of two ova.

Binovular twins These are often referred to as non-identical or dizygotic twins. The
(dizygotic) tendency for a woman to produce more than one ovum each month is inclined to be hereditary, unless drug-induced. These twins therefore tend to be familial. Each ovum is fertilised by a different sperm and the twins may therefore be of the same, or of different sexes and are no more alike than any other two siblings. In the uterus, they each have their own placenta, amnion and chorionic sac.

Uniovular twins Such twins are really an abnormal occurrence. Fertilisation of an
(monozygotic) ovum takes place in the normal way but the zygote divides into two, resulting in two cells, each with a nucleus containing identical chromosome patterns. These twins are often referred to as identical or monozygotic twins, being alike in every way. In the uterus they share the same placenta.

The actual stage at which the zygote divides seems to vary. Sometimes it is believed to occur after formation of the amniotic sac so that the twins even share the same amnion. Because this is not a

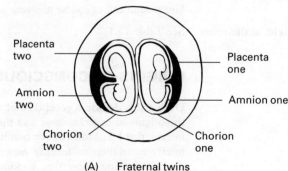

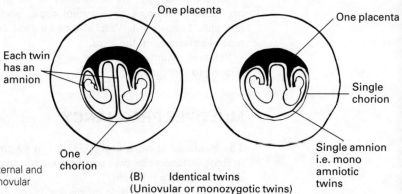

Fig. 14.4A & B Fraternal and identical twins (A) Binovular (B) Uniovular

normal occurrence, one or both twins are more likely in this case to have a congenital abnormality. Siamese, or conjoined, twins are of course uniovular.

ASSESSMENT OF FETAL WELL-BEING

Antenatal booking visit Accurate and fully detailed history-taking at the first antenatal visit is a valuable means of identifying many factors which put the fetus at risk. The following facts should be elicited:

Maternal age The optimum age for childbearing is between the mother's 18th and 35th birthdays, the optimum maximum age for a primigravida being lowered to 30.

Family medical history 1. *Multiple pregnancy* which has not occurred in association with the administration of drugs for infertility.
2. *Allergic conditions* such as asthma or eczema.
3. *Genetically-inherited diseases* which may be:
   a. sex-linked
   b. race-linked
   c. transmitted by dominant or recessive genes.

There is an increased risk of genetically-inherited disease if a child's parents are closely related.

4. *Infectious diseases* which may be transmitted to those living in close contact, e.g. tuberculosis.

Mother's own medical history

1. Any medical condition which is likely to reduce oxygenation and nourishment to the fetus, e.g. essential hypertension, cardiac conditions, severe anaemia, unstable diabetes.
2. Smoking, alcohol or drug addiction.
3. All drugs taken from the time of conception must be recorded since they may be detrimental to fetal well-being.

Mother's social background

The social class of a married woman is based on her husband's occupation, that of the single woman upon her own occupation and that of the single girl who is a minor on the occupation of her father.

It is a well-documented fact that the lower the social class the higher the perinatal and infant mortality rates, but it must also be remembered that social class is not always linked with level of income, although it may be linked with a way of life.

Social factors do have an enormous influence on health and well-being and, where poor housing, overcrowding, a lack of basic amenities and an inadequate or unbalanced diet exist, the stress factors which they induce inevitably have an unfavourable effect upon the fetus.

Yet again, a frightened schoolgirl who conceals her pregnancy in fear of parental disapprobation, or the overburdened multiparous woman with yet another unwanted infant on the way, are certainly not able to convey to the fetus in utero that bonding of love which is so essential to his well-being.

Menstrual history

It is useful to know at what age a mother started to menstruate, whether her periods are normal and regular and the length of the cycle. This gives some guide to her fertility and hormone balance.

The first day of the last menstrual period is noted so that the expected date of delivery can be estimated. This date is useful in assessing the duration of pregnancy in relation to the size of the uterus throughout pregnancy.

Previous obstetric history

The following details need to be recorded because they help to identify problems which could affect the current pregnancy:

1. Previous spontaneous or therapeutic abortions
2. Previous complications of pregnancy, labour and puerperium
3. Duration of previous pregnancies
4. Weight and condition at birth of previous infants.

During the course of pregnancy

Fetal well-being can be assessed as pregnancy advances also by keeping the following records:

Maternal weight gain

This should be in relation to the period of pregnancy.

In the first half of pregnancy the approximate weight gain is 2 kg. In the second half of pregnancy there is an average gain of 0.5 kg per week.

Excessive weight gain or weight loss should always be investigated.

Abdominal palpation The height of the fundus should relate to the estimated weeks of pregnancy. If they do not relate and there is also either an excessive weight gain or an excessive weight loss, then multiple pregnancy or hydramnios may be the cause of excessive weight gain and intrauterine retarded growth or intrauterine death may be related to weight loss. But 'dates' and the period of pregnancy must also be checked.

Ultrasound scan *In the first trimester* it is possible to identify the embryonic sac or sacs and fetal heart movements. Crown to rump measurements and fetal skull measurements can be made.

In the second trimester scanning is usually carried out routinely at 16–18 weeks. In addition to the above findings, the abdominal circumference gives an assessment of liver size and the length of the femur can be recorded.

In the presence of suspected intrauterine retarded growth serial measurements can be made to assess development of the fetus, and for mothers at risk the following measurements are recorded every 2 weeks after the 30th week of pregnancy.

- Biparietal diameter
- Abdominal circumference
- Ratio between head and abdominal circumference
- Placental localisation
- Volume of amniotic fluid

For further details regarding ultrasound scanning see page 206.

Kick charts The mother may be asked to keep a record of fetal movements by completing a daily kick chart. About 10 movements during the same 12-hour period is an average pattern. Excessive fetal movements and fewer movements are both indications of fetal hypoxia. Cessation of movements entirely suggests intrauterine death. The mother is asked to report to the hospital if the normal pattern changes significantly. Fetal movements may also be felt by a midwife's hands when she is palpating the mother's abdomen. It is also possible to see fetal movements on the mother's abdomen after the middle trimester.

Fetal heart As well as recording the fetal heart by sonic means, it can be heard with a stethoscope after the 20th week of pregnancy. The normal rate is 120–160 beats per minute. Further investigations, which are carried out primarily to exclude fetal or placental abnormalities, are described on page 204.

Biophysical profiles These were introduced by Manning in 1981. The examination is carried out towards the end of pregnancy. The mother has an ultrasound scan lasting 30–40 minutes and cardiotocograph apparatus is used to carry out a 20-minute trace of the fetal heart.

Table 14.2 Biophysical profiles (a modified scheme)

Event	Score 2	Score 0
1. Fetal breathing movements	>30 s of sustained FBM	<30 s of FBM in 30 mins
2. Fetal body movements	3 gross movements	<3 gross movements in 30 mins
3. Fetal limb movements	Flexion/extension	no flexion
4. Fetal heart reactivity	2 accelerations in 15 secs	<2 accelerations in 40 mins
5. Amniotic fluid volume	1 cm pocket of fluid in 2 perpendicular planes	<1 cm pocket of fluid

Examination can last up to 40 min
Score 8–10 repeat in 1 week
Score 4–6 deliver if mature/otherwise repeat daily
Score 0–2 indicates necessity for immediate delivery
> = more than < = less than

CHROMOSOMAL AND GENETICALLY-INHERITED CONDITIONS

Non-disjunction When the nucleus of a cell divides, the chromosomes separate longitudinally so that the pairs are divided into two identical sets. Occasionally one pair of chromosomes fails to separate so that while one daughter cell carries an undivided pair of chromosomes, the other has a missing chromosome.

At fertilisation, one chromosome from the other partner combines with the undivided pair in that cell to form a **trisomy**. The second daughter cell with the missing chromosome usually fails to survive.

Down's syndrome is the commonest type of abnormality arising from disjunction, a trisomy of the 21st pair having occurred.

Turner's syndrome is the commonest abnormality which arises when the daughter cell containing the missing chromosome continues to develop instead of failing to survive.

Inherited characteristics
(Fig. 14.5A & B) Blood groups can be used here as an example to show how the child's own group is determined. Taking a mother who is AA homozygous and a father who is AB heterozygous, any of the combinations given in Figure 14.5A is possible.

If both parents are AB heterozygous then the situation is as given in Figure 14.5B.

Dominantly-inherited disease
(Fig. 14.6) Only one parent need have a dominant gene for this type of inherited disease to occur. The most well known diseases transmitted in this way are **achondroplasia**, **Huntington's chorea** and **osteogenesis imperfecta**.

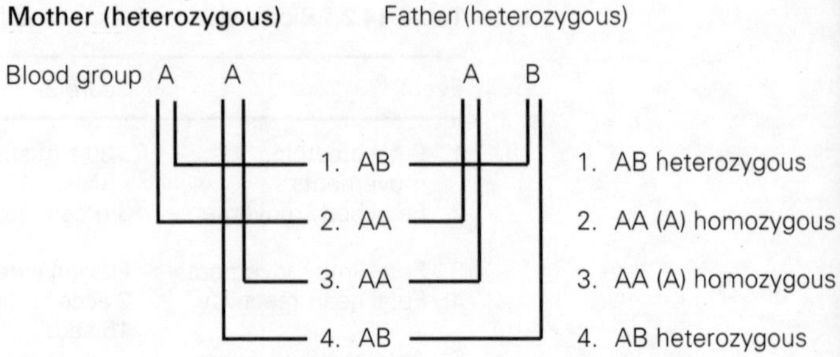

Mother (heterozygous)   Father (heterozygous)

Blood group A   A   A   B

1. AB — 1. AB heterozygous
2. AA — 2. AA (A) homozygous
3. AA — 3. AA (A) homozygous
4. AB — 4. AB heterozygous

Fig. 14.5A Combinations possible when one parent is AB heterozygous.

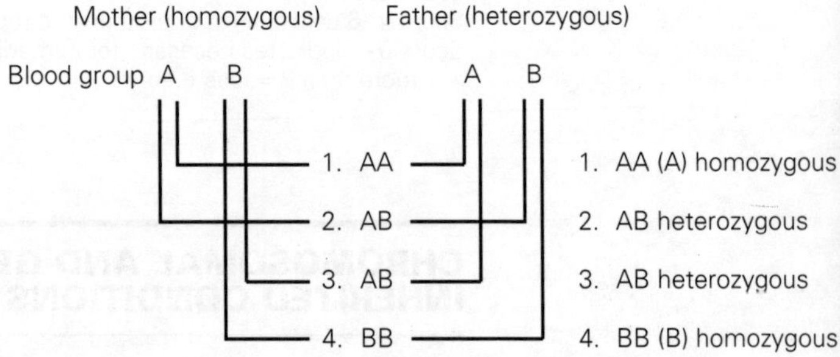

Mother (homozygous)   Father (heterozygous)

Blood group A   B   A   B

1. AA — 1. AA (A) homozygous
2. AB — 2. AB heterozygous
3. AB — 3. AB heterozygous
4. BB — 4. BB (B) homozygous

Fig. 14.5B Combinations possible when both parents are AB heterozygous.

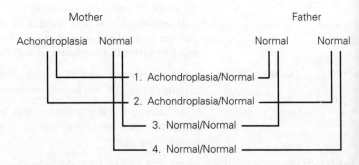

Mother   Father

Achondroplasia   Normal   Normal   Normal

1. Achondroplasia/Normal
2. Achondroplasia/Normal
3. Normal/Normal
4. Normal/Normal

Fig. 14.6 Patterns of dominant inheritance.

Children 1 and 2 in this diagram inherit achondroplasia. Children 3 and 4 are unaffected.

Recessively-inherited disease If we take normal healthy parents who each have a disease such as
(Fig. 14.7A, B) cystic fibrosis on a recessive gene, the probability of inheritance is greater than if only one parent carries it although if a male inherits cystic fibrosis, he is likely to be sterile.

Sex-linked genetic inheritance Sometimes a gene is linked to a sex-determining chromosome and
(Fig. 14.8A, B) disease is transmitted by an X or Y chromosome. The defective gene carrying haemophilia is carried on the X chromosome.

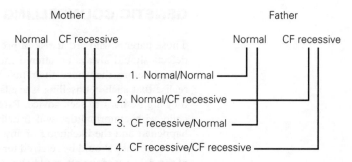

Fig. 14.7A Recessively-inherited disease. Recessive inheritance – both parents carry cystic fibrosis on a recessive gene

In this example:
The 1st child will not be affected at all.
The 2nd and 3rd will carry the recessive CF gene.
The 4th child will inherit the disease.

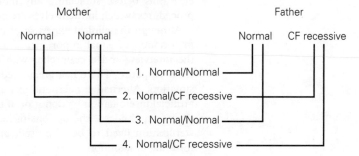

Fig. 14.7B Recessive inheritance – one parent carries cystic fibrosis (CF) on a recessive gene.

In this example:
The 1st and 3rd children will not be affected at all.
The 2nd and 4th will both be carriers of cystic fibrosis.

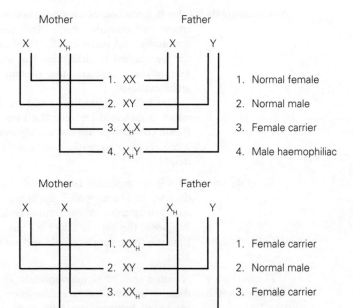

Fig. 14.8A Sex-linked inheritance. Offspring of a healthy mother who carries haemophilia and a normal father. the gene carrying haemophilia is carried on the X chromosome and the disease is transmitted only to the male.

Fig. 14.8B If the mother is normal but father is a haemophiliac.

GENETIC COUNSELLING

Those parents who are at risk of producing a child with congenital defects should always be offered the opportunity of genetic counselling before they have their first baby. Some parents may not realise that such counselling is available, others are so anxious that they are hesitant to seek advice. Parents who have already had one child with abnormalities will usually be anxious to know why it happened and the likelihood of any future children being similarly affected. They should be referred for counselling within a short time of the delivery of the affected baby.

There are some parents who will seek advice but who are prepared to embark upon parenthood and then to continue with the pregnancy even if fetal abnormality is diagnosed. It is as well to elicit this before subjecting any mother to unwanted diagnostic procedures, which in themselves are not without risk to the fetus.

Although the clinical expertise of the geneticist is of the utmost importance, of equal importance is a non-clinical environment for the interview and a counsellor who can communicate easily and show empathy. There is a great need to reduce the tension of the situation. Alternative decisions to normal pregnancy may include artificial insemination by donor or, if the parents decide not to have their own children, the options of long-term contraception versus sterilisation need to be discussed, and perhaps the possibility of fostering or adoption.

DIAGNOSIS OF FETAL ABNORMALITY

Amniocentesis

This is a method of obtaining amniotic fluid by introducing a fine trocar and cannula (sterile) into the amniotic cavity through the abdominal and uterine walls. Fetal cells are shed into the fluid and can be studied to determine the sex and well-being of the fetus. For obvious reasons, the placenta must be located prior to amniocentesis.

The following studies would be made on a specimen of fluid which is aspirated between the 14th and 18th weeks of pregnancy. Results of analysis are not usually available for at least 3 weeks and more recent diagnostic tests have been designed to obviate this delay.

Sex of the fetus

This is an important factor where there is a possibility of sex-linked disease, e.g. haemophilia, for the question of termination of pregnancy may arise. Where amniocentesis is used as the means of diagnosis, the mother may have already felt fetal movements by the time the results are available and emotional conflict is then likely to arise.

The presence of alphafetoprotein

A raised level of alphafetoprotein in the amniotic fluid may be indicative of spina bifida and/or anencephaly and is most accurately estimated between the 16th and 18th weeks of pregnancy. The amount of alphafetoprotein in the amniotic fluid is a more accurate indication of neural-tube defects than that in maternal serum but it is by no means a positive indication. An ultrasound scan in the second trimester will also confirm or exclude the condition.

Chromosome studies can determine such conditions as Down's syndrome, Turner's syndrome and Klinefelter's syndrome. The same studies can now be carried out in the first trimester by chorionic villus biopsy and the results are available almost immediately.

Haemolytic disease This is now rarely seen in the UK but where it is suspected a specimen of amniotic fluid might be obtained to assess its severity. The procedure would also be carried out to treat the condition and allow the administration of an intraperitoneal blood transfusion to the fetus.

Lung function tests This is not a test to diagnose congenital abnormality but it is carried out in the last trimester of pregnancy where labour is to be induced or caesarean section carried out before full term. It is dependent upon the ratio of lipids (lecithin and sphingomyelin) in the amniotic fluid and amniocentesis must therefore be carried out. Lipids enable the alveoli of the lungs to expand when the infant takes his first breath and to continue this movement once respiration is established. The lipids are produced from the middle of pregnancy onwards and lecithin is produced in greater amounts after the 34th week.

Fetoscopy This diagnostic technique involves examination of the fetus through the mother's abdominal wall with the use of a fibre-optic telescope. It can be performed under either local or general anaesthesia. It should be preceded by ultrasound scan in order to determine the period of gestation. If fetal blood is required, the examination should be carried out at 18–20 weeks while the amniotic fluid is still clear. Blood for haematology can be examined for such conditions as thalassaemia, sickle-cell disease, Duchenne muscular dystrophy and haemophilia. Results are available the same day, whereas the culture of cells obtained via amniocentesis may take 3 weeks. Fetal skin samples can also be obtained rather than the desquamated cells obtained from the amniotic fluid.

The entire fetus can be viewed at 16–17 weeks of gestation when the amniotic fluid is clear and the fetus still small. Later than this, the scanner used in conjunction with fetoscopy helps to guide the fetoscope to the area to be viewed. Conditions such as a low spina bifida, limb deformities, hare lip and cleft palate can be diagnosed by this means – conditions that ultrasound and X-ray would not reveal.

Chorionic villus biopsy Chorionic villus biopsy has the advantage of being possible in the first trimester and of giving results almost immediately. This is an advantage at a time when there is a growing demand for the earliest possible diagnosis of fetal abnormality. It also avoids the unhappy situation in which a mother who has already felt fetal movements must decide whether or not to have her pregnancy terminated.

On the other hand, recent studies are beginning to link the occurrence of fetal limb deformities with chorionic villus sampling done at this early stage.

Ultrasound is used to guide a cannula through the cervix to where chorionic villi are most profuse and villi are then extracted either by vacuum extraction or an endoscopic biopsy is carried out. The cells of the trophoblast, being part of the zygote, have the same genetic make-up as the fetus. The tissue obtained can therefore be used for chromosome, DNA and biochemical analysis and because the sex of the fetus is determined, sex-linked diseases can be excluded or confirmed. Metabolic disorders where the relative enzyme is absent can also be detected.

Ultrasound scan   Although there was some controversy concerning the use of ultrasound diagnostic procedures at the National Institute of Health Conference in 1984, the Royal College of Obstetrics and Gynaecologists recommended that it be used routinely in pregnancy at 16–18 weeks. There is no evidence to suggest that the procedure is hazardous to either mother or fetus but it was recommended that machines should be operated with the lowest exposure. During pregnancy it can be used as follows:

In the first trimester

5 weeks	the embryonic sac can be identified
6–7 weeks	fetal heart movements can be seen
7 weeks	twins can be diagnosed by the identification of two amniotic sacs
7–14 weeks	crown to rump measurement can be recorded and maturity accurately determined
13–14 weeks	fetal head can be identified and measured.

Ultrasound might also be used in these early weeks prior to chorion biopsy or fetoscopy when those tests need to be made, or when serial measurements of the BP diameter of the skull are to be recorded.

In the second trimester   it is used as a routine investigation at 16–18 weeks unless the mother prefers not to have the procedure carried out. It is used to:

1. Establish the gestational period by estimating:
   - crown to rump measurement
   - fetal skull measurements
   - biparietal diameter
   - head circumference
   - abdominal circumference
     to assess size of liver
   - length of femur
2. Diagnose multiple pregnancy
3. Identify hydatidiform or carneous mole
4. Identify some fetal abnormalities – anencephaly, hydrocephaly, spina bifida
5. Locate the placenta and therefore diagnose placenta praevia

It may be used additionally at this time to identify the position of the fetus and placenta prior to amniocentesis or fetoscopy.

In the last trimester it is used to:

1. Identify fetal respiratory movements (these movements are for exercise only – oxygen and carbon dioxide are exchanged via the placenta)
2. Exclude fetal abnormalities (as above) and intrauterine death
3. Diagnose malpresentations
4. Diagnose placenta praevia
5. Diagnose hydramnios
6. Assess maternal pelvis and fetal skull measurements and exclude disproportion.

It is also used after the 32nd week of pregnancy to make serial measurements in the presence of intrauterine retarded growth. The biparietal diameter should increase by 0.15–0.2 cm per week and this provides a satisfactory estimate of growth. Ultrasonography provides almost immediate estimates whereas serial urinary oestriol levels are much less reliable. It takes 24 hours to produce a urine sample and there is then a further time lapse for laboratory estimations to be carried out.

Cordocentesis This is now being introduced in many obstetric units because, while it can detect chromosome, metabolic and blood disorders, it is a simpler procedure than amniocentesis and entails less risk. Using ultrasound to determine placental position and using the maternal transabdominal route, a fine gauge needle is guided to the base of the umbilical cord and blood is withdrawn from a fetal vessel.

X-ray examination This is now a much less popular method of diagnosis because of the proven effects that radiation has on the maternal ovaries and developing fetus. Leukaemia and genetic mutation have been associated with its use and ultrasound scanning is now used in preference. If a pregnant woman does require an X-ray because ultrasound is not available, it should be postponed until after the 32nd week of pregnancy. Nor should a woman of childbearing years be X-rayed during the postovulatory phase of the menstrual cycle if there is any possibility that she might have conceived.

The greatest hazards of exposure to radiation are leukaemia and genetic mutation. The latter may persist over several generations. Where X-ray examination is still practised it may be used:

1. *To assess the measurements of the mother's pelvis in relation to the size of the fetal skull* to exclude disproportion. This would be done after 36 weeks if the fetal head could not be made to engage.
2. *To diagnose malpresentation at term* but before the commencement of labour.
3. *To confirm multiple pregnancy*. This could be delayed until the 32nd week.
4. *To confirm intrauterine death* when no fetal movements have been felt, no fetal heart can be heard and a decision needs to be made regarding the induction of labour. Fetal death is confirmed by

overlapping of the skull bones, known as Spalding's sign, and the presence of gas in the major blood vessels.

DEALING WITH FETAL ABNORMALITY

When fetal abnormality has been diagnosed it is important that the parents, after sympathetic counselling, should be given a little time to make their own decision about termination of pregnancy and that pressure should not be brought to bear upon them by relatives or professionals.

Although the bearing and rearing of a child with congenital abnormalities brings its own stresses to the parents, these stresses are not always greater than the long-term psychological traumas with which termination of pregnancy is sometimes associated.

It is also an established fact that some children who were diagnosed as having fetal abnormalities have been perfectly healthy at birth – and vice versa.

DEVELOPMENT OF AMNION AND AMNIOTIC FLUID

AMNIOTIC MEMBRANE (Fig. 14.2B, C, D)

The amniotic membrane is derived from the ectoderm which lined the amniotic cavity. As the developing fetus enlarges, so the amniotic cavity is pushed further and further outwards until the cavity of the uterus is filled. (Simultaneously, as already stated, this is when the decidua capsularis is pushed outwards to lie against the decidua vera and the chorionic membrane is formed as the villi atrophy.) At this stage, therefore, the uterus is lined with chorion and the amnion forming the fetal sac lies within the chorionic membrane and covers the cord, or body stalk, which connects the fetus with the developing placenta.

The amnion at term is a thin and transparent, but very tough membrane which can be stripped away from the chorion to the area of the cord insertion. It continues to cover it for the entire length and is then continuous with fetal skin at the umbilicus.

AMNIOTIC FLUID

The increasing size of the amniotic cavity is due partly to the developing fetus and partly to the presence of the fluid which appears from the 4th week of pregnancy. It is derived largely from the cells of the amniotic membrane, the ectoderm. Fetal urine is found in the amniotic fluid from as early as the 14th week, the urine being mostly water, since waste products are excreted via the fetal/maternal circulatory systems. After 20 weeks fluid from the fetal lungs is also passed into it.

The fluid, sometimes called **liquor amnii**, is a clear, straw-coloured fluid with an alkaline reaction and can therefore be distinguished from maternal urine following the rupture of membranes. The amount produced increases throughout pregnancy so that by the 38th week there is about 1 litre contained in the amniotic sac. After the 28th week the volume diminishes. The fetus swallows about 400 ml every day and there is a gradual change of fluid about every 3 hours.

Composition

99% water 1% solids. The solids include:

Protein	Urea
Fat	Uric acid
Carbohydrate	Bile pigments
Mineral salts	Vernix caseosa
Enzymes	Lanugo
Placental hormones	Desquamated fetal cells

Functions

1. Allows the fetus free movement
2. Enables fetal limbs to develop and move without being compressed by each other, the fetal trunk or the walls of the uterus.
3. Equalises intrauterine pressure and acts as a shock absorber.
4. Stabilises intrauterine temperature.

In labour, providing that the sac of fluid remains intact until labour is well advanced, it:

1. Acts as a cushion to protect the fetal head from pressure
2. Maintains a sterile environment for the fetus
3. Acts as a wedge to aid dilatation of the cervix
4. Reduces the effect of uterine contractions of the placental circulation
5. Provides the birth canal with a sterile douche immediately prior to delivery when the amniotic sac is ruptured.

Abnormalities of amniotic fluid

Polyhydramnios

This is an excessive amount of amniotic fluid which is associated with maternal diabetes, neural-tube defects and oesophageal atresia in the fetus and uniovular twins. Malpresentation of the fetus and unstable lie are both commonly associated with the condition and prolapse of the umbilical cord is more likely to occur.

Oligohydramnios

describes a diminished amount of amniotic fluid which does not allow adequate fetal movement in utero. In some instances the fetal limbs are so compressed that the mother needs to be taught how to stimulate the infant's movements following delivery. His skin is dry and leathery in appearance. Oligohydramnios is also associated with the very rare condition of renal agenesis.

Colour
1. Meconium staining gives the liquor a greenish-brown tinge and is a sign of fetal distress
2. Bile-stained liquor is an indication of haemolytic disease but is now rarely seen in the UK

THE FETAL CIRCULATION

Before the fetal circulation can be fully understood, the general structures and principles of the adult circulation must be brought to mind.

The adult circulatory system

Venous blood from the lower limbs is returned to the right auricle of the heart by the inferior vena cava, and venous blood from the upper extremities is returned to the right auricle by the superior vena cava. From the right auricle, blood passes through the tricuspid valve to the right ventricle and is then pumped to the lungs for replenishment of oxygen by the pulmonary artery. Four pulmonary veins take the newly oxygenated blood from the lungs to the left auricle of the heart, where it passes through the mitral valve into the left ventricle.

From the left ventricle, the aorta sends blood into two streams: the ascending branch supplies the head and upper limbs, the descending branch supplies all parts of the body below the level of the diaphragm. Following its circulation to upper and lower extremities, the blood is again returned to the heart by the superior and inferior vena cava.

During intrauterine life, the lungs of the fetus are inactive and interchange of oxygen and carbon dioxide takes place through the placenta. Extra structures are therefore present in the fetal circulatory system which become useless once the extrauterine function of respiration is established.

Additional structures in the fetal circulation
(Fig. 14.9)

1. Umbilical vein

carries oxygenated blood from the placenta to the undersurface of the liver.

2. Ductus venosus

leaves the umbilical vein before it reaches the liver and transmits the greater part of the newly oxygenated blood into the inferior vena cava, so bypassing the liver.

3. Foramen ovale

is an opening which allows blood to pass from the right auricle into the left auricle.

4. Ductus arteriosus

is a bypass extending between the right ventricle and the descending aorta.

5. Hypogastric arteries

are two vessels which return blood from the fetus to the placenta. In the umbilical cord they are known as umbilical arteries. Inside the fetus they are known as hypogastric arteries.

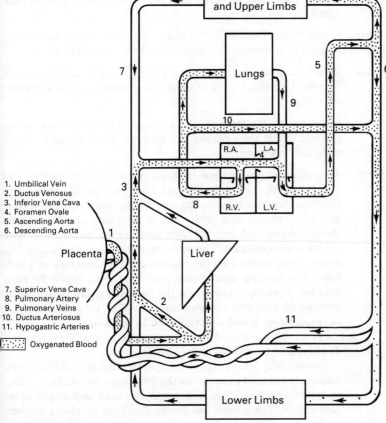

1. Umbilical Vein
2. Ductus Venosus
3. Inferior Vena Cava
4. Foramen Ovale
5. Ascending Aorta
6. Descending Aorta

7. Superior Vena Cava
8. Pulmonary Artery
9. Pulmonary Veins
10. Ductus Arteriosus
11. Hypogastric Arteries

Oxygenated Blood

Fig. 14.9 Fetal circulation.

Fetal circulatory system

Umbilical vein   carries blood, rich in oxygen, from the placenta to the undersurface of the liver. The hepatic vein leaves the liver and returns blood to the inferior vena cava.

Ductus venosus   branches from the umbilical vein and transmits the greater amount of oxygenated blood into the inferior vena cava.

Inferior vena cava,   already transmitting blood which has circulated in the fetal lower limbs and trunk, receives blood from the hepatic vein and ductus venosus and takes it to the right auricle of the heart.

Foramen ovale   allows the greater part of the oxygenated blood in the right auricle to pass on to the left auricle, from where it is passed through the mitral valve to the left ventricle and then through the aorta into its ascending branch to supply the head and upper extremities. It can be seen, therefore, that the liver, heart and brain receive the best supply of the newly oxygenated blood.

Superior vena cava   returns blood from the head and upper extremities to the right auricle. This, with the remainder of the stream brought in by the inferior vena cava, passes through the tricuspid valve into the right ventricle.

Pulmonary artery   shunts some of this supply of mixed blood to the non-functioning lungs, which fortunately require only a little nourishment

Ductus arteriosus   shunts the greater part of the blood from the right ventricle directly into the descending aorta to supply the abdomen, pelvis and lower extremities.

Hypogastric arteries,   extensions of the internal iliac arteries, carry blood back to the placenta where more oxygen and nutrients are supplied from the maternal circulation.

Changes at birth   *The infant cries and expands his lungs,* causing an increased flow of blood through the four pulmonary veins into the left auricle and equalising pressure between the right and left auricles. The pressure in the left auricle rises while that in the pulmonary artery falls. Blood is drawn back from the aorta along the ductus arteriosus until the lungs are expanded. The pressure in the inferior vena cava falls when venous return from the placenta ceases. There may be a little blood flow from the inferior vena cava into the left auricle for a few days but it gradually ceases and the **foramen ovale closes** as the pressure on right and left sides equalises. With the **establishment of respiration, blood is oxygenated in the lungs**.

The umbilical cord ceases to conduct oxygenated blood to the fetus and deoxygenated blood back to the placenta.

The umbilical arteries close more quickly than the umbilical vein which allows blood to return to the fetus from the placenta. Many midwives therefore refrain from cutting the cord until all pulsations have ceased. The arteries will fibrose distally to become a supporting ligament of the bladder.

The umbilical vein fibroses to become a supporting ligament of the liver.

The first few centimetres of the *hypogastric arteries* remain patent and are retained as the interior iliac arteries.

The ductus venosus fibroses and becomes a ligament supporting the liver.

The ductus arteriosus contracts as the lungs expand because blood now passes it by. It does not always close immediately but gradually fibroses to become a cardiac ligament.

By the end of the first week of neonatal life the fetal end of the cord should have dried and separated from the skin of the infant.

Respiration at birth is irregular, with short periods of apnoea, the rate of respiration being about 50 per minute. Abdominal muscle movement is very evident. The respiration rate settles within a short space of time to 40 per minute.

Summary

Extra structures in fetal   ● umbilical vein
circulation   ● ductus venosus

- foramen ovale
- ductus arteriosus
- hypogastric arteries

Initiation of respiration effected by

1. Stimulation of respiratory centre by rising carbon dioxide levels
2. External sensory stimulus lowered
   - temperature of environment
   - light
   - sound
   - touch
   - body is no longer weightless

Changes at birth

1. Cessation of placental blood supply
2. Expansion and aeration of lungs
3. Closure of foramen ovale
4. Fibrosis of:
   - umbilical vein
   - ductus venosus
   - hypogastric arteries
   - ductus arteriosus

Aeration of alveoli

The primitive heart, lungs and circulatory system are established by the end of the 3rd week of gestation and, by the end of the 4th week, blood is circulating through them. Fetal heart movements can be seen on ultrasound scan in the 6th week of intrauterine life and, in the last trimester, fetal respiratory movements can be identified. These respiratory movements, which originated earlier in pregnancy, encourage the movement of amniotic fluid into the respiratory tract so that not only the airways, but also the alveoli, are filled with fluid.

Most of this fluid is expelled during delivery when the thorax becomes compressed as it descends through the birth canal. It is essential, however, that the infant's airways are aspirated before he takes his first breath, otherwise he will inhale any fluid that remains there as well as fragments of vernix, lanugo, meconium and blood. Should such inhalation occur, the right bronchus is more likely to be obstructed than the left because the right has a more vertical position.

Aeration and expansion of the alveoli is considerably more involved than simply the establishing of respiratory muscle movement. Not only the elastic resistance of the tissues, but also the surface tension of fluid lining the alveoli has to be overcome. Therefore, a much higher negative pressure than that required for aeration during normal respiratory movement is needed. The process is aided by a **surfactant** (the lipids lecithin and sphingomyelin) which is produced in the lungs from about the 24th week of pregnancy. By its detergent action it helps to dissolve the film of fluid which lines the alveoli and thereby facilitates the interchange of oxygen and carbon dioxide. It also prevents the alveoli from collapsing again during normal respiratory movement. Full expansion of the lungs is not immediate but has usually occurred by the 4th day of life.

Before the 28th week of pregnancy there is very little surfactant and this, together with the immaturity of the alveoli and pulmonary circulation, gives a poor prognosis for the survival of an infant born so prematurely. The efficiency of surfactant can be assessed at fetoscopy if a decision must be made to terminate pregnancy prematurely. This gives some indication as to whether induction of labour should be delayed in the interests of the fetus. A deficiency of surfactant is associated with respiratory distress syndrome. The lungs at birth have only about one-sixth of the alveoli that will eventually be required and growth and proliferation of these tissues continue until the eighth year of life.

Stimulation of the respiratory centre

Because the fetal lungs are not functional during intrauterine life, the interchange of oxygen and carbon dioxide is effected through the placenta.

To aid oxygenation of his tissues the fetus has a high red blood-cell count and therefore a high level of fetal haemoglobin. This compensates for the 'mixed' blood which is transmitted in the fetal blood vessels. At about the 36th week of intrauterine life, fetal haemoglobin begins to fall. Then during labour there is a 30% decrease in oxygenation when uterine contractions diminish the blood flow to the fetus. During the second stage of labour, rising carbon dioxide levels in the fetal circulatory system stimulate the respiratory centre in the medulla and at birth, external stimuli of temperature, touch and light all play an important part in his first inspiration. His initial gasps are almost immediately followed by the typical loud wail of a newly-born infant as his lungs are expanded. His abdominal muscles are brought into play as the diaphragm and intercostal muscles attempt to fully expand the thoracic cavity.

Should carbon dioxide levels rise excessively before delivery is imminent, fetal distress becomes evident and, unless immediate steps are taken, the respiratory centre is depressed instead of being stimulated. Should carbon dioxide levels just reach the point of stimulating respiration while the fetus is still in the uterus, his gasp for breath will include inhalation of amniotic fluid and any solids that it contains. Fetal distress will develop, his delivery must be expedited and a paediatrician should be present at delivery.

When the apparently fluid-filled lungs of a stillborn infant are placed in a tank of water at postmortem examination, they sink because there has been no aeration. Should they float, then some aeration must have occurred and the infant was not stillborn.

REVISION QUESTIONS

State two advantages to the embryo which result from the separation of his blood from his mother's.
Of what importance to the fetus are the following:
amniotic fluid
umbilical cord
uterine muscle.

What is the physiological effect on the fetus of a uterine contraction?
State and explain one factor which causes:

the newborn baby to breathe
the newborn baby to cry.

Why does the newborn infant use abdominal muscles in respiration?
What anatomical change occurs in the heart when a newborn infant takes his first breath?
Give the average length, weight, and head circumference of a newborn infant.
What hormone is released by the pituitary after the placenta has been expelled? What is its function?
How is the newborn infant's neuromuscular system assessed?

REFERENCES AND FURTHER READING

Books and reports
Annis L F 1978 Child before birth. Cornell University Press, New York
Berrill N J 1969 The person in the womb. Dodd Mead, London
Cameron N 1990 Is life really sacred? Kingsway, Eastbourne
Dryden R 1978 Before birth. Heinemann, London
England M A 1983 A colour atlas of life before birth: normal fetal development. Wolfe Medical, London
Fitzsimmons J S 1980 A handbook of clinical genetics. Heinemann Medical, London
Heddell F 1980 Accident of birth: aspects of mental handicap. BBC Publications, London
Joffe J M 1969 Pre-natal determinants of behaviour. Penguin, Harmondsworth
Kuhse H, Singer P 1985 Should the baby live?: the problem of handicapped infants. Oxford University Press, Oxford
MacNutt F, MacNutt J 1988 Praying for your unborn child. Hodder & Stoughton, London
Milunsky A 1980 Know your genes. Penguin, Harmondsworth
Moore K L 1983 Before we are born: basic embryology and birth defects. W B Saunders, Philadelphia
Newman G, Eareckson J 1987 All God's children: ministry to the disabled. Marshall-Pickering, Basingstoke
Nilsson L 1967 The everyday miracle: a child is born. Allen Lane, London
Roberts D, Thomson A 1976 The biology of fetal growth. Symposium of the Society for the Study of Human Biology
Rugh R, Shettles L 1971 From conception to birth: the drama of life's beginnings. Harper & Row, New York
Sadow J L D 1980 Human reproduction: an integrated view. Croom Helm, London

Smith D W 1979 Mothering your unborn baby. W B Saunders, Philadelphia

Tanner J M 1978 Foetus into man: physical growth from conception to maturity. Castlemead, Ware

Verney T, Kelly T 1987 Silent world of the unborn child. Sphere Books, London

Articles

Abramovitch D, Page K 1987 Fetal control of amniotic fluid. Contemporary Reviews in Obstetrics and Gynaecology 1(4): 241–248

Anon 1989 Kick charts may alarm. Nursing Times 85: 9

Bastide A, Manning F, Harman C, Lange I, Morrison I 1986 Ultrasound evaluation of amniotic fluid: outcome of pregnancies with severe oligohydramnios. American Journal of Obstetrics and Gynecology 154(4): 895–900

Benacerraf BR, Gatter M A, Ginsburgh F 1984 Ultrasound diagnosis of meconium-stained amniotic fluid. American Journal of Obstetrics and Gynecology 149(5): 570–572

Bowley A 1989 Midwives and ultrasound. Midwives' Chronicle 102: 87

Brace R, Wolf E 1989 Normal amniotic fluid changes throughout pregnancy. American Journal of Obstetrics and Gynecology 16(2): 383–387

Brambati B 1987 Chorionic villus sampling IPPF Research in Reproduction (April): 1–2

Brumfield C et al 1987 Amniotic fluid: alphafetoprotein levels and pregnancy outcome. British Journal of Obstetrics and Gynaecology 157(4): 822–825

Davies L 1987 Daily fetal movement counting: a valuable assessment tool. Journal of Nursing and Midwifery 32: 11–19

Dudley N J, Lamb M P, Copping C 1987 A new method for fetal weight estimation using real-time ultrasound. British Journal of Obstetrics and Gynaecology 94(2): 110–114

Eden R D, Seifert L S, Kodack L D, Trofatter K F, Killam A P, Gall S A 1988 A modified biophysical profile for antenatal fetal surveillance. Obstetrics and Gynecology 71 (3 Pt 1): 365–369

Fry J 1985 Ultrasound scanning in pregnancy. Update (15 July): 101

Furness M E 1987 Reporting obstetric ultrasound. Lancet i: 675–676

Gegor C et al 1991 Antepartum fetal assessment: a nurse/midwifery perspective. Journal of Nursing and Midwifery 36(3): 837–839

Grant A 1986 Controlled trials of routine ultrasound in pregnancy. Birth 13: 22–28

Hill L M, Breckle R, Wolfgram K R, O'Brien P C 1983 Oligohydramnios: ultrasonically detected incidence and subsequent fetal outcome. American Journal of Obstetrics and Gynecology 147(4): 407–410

Heam I 1990 Fetal monitoring: current practice in England and Wales. Journal of Obstetrics and Gynaecology (April): 281–285

James D 1991 Limitations of biophysical profiles. Contemporary Reviews in Obstetrics and Gynaecology 3(2): 69–73

Jones D G 1989 Brain birth and personal identity. Journal of Medical Ethics 15(4): 173–178

Kenyon S 1989 Making a game of obstetric ultrasound. Nursing Times (2 August): 39–41

Kenyon S 1985 Obstetric scanning: the midwife's involvement. Nursing Times? (19 July): 52–55

Kenyon S 1989 Obstetric ultrasound. Midwife, Health Visitor and Community Nurse (June): 246–251

Lennox C et al 1988 Ultrasound screening in the mid trimester of pregnancy: identification of multiple pregnancy and fetal abnormality and pregnancies resulting in mid trimester loss. British Journal of Obstetrics and Gynaecology 9(2): 87–89

Liley A 1972 The fetus as a personality. Australian and New Zealand

Journal of Psychology 6: 99

Livingstone A 1991 Fetal circulation: a continuing problem in Britain. British Medical Journal (23 Feb): 497–498

Meade T, Grant A 1987 Early amniocentesis: a cytogenic evaluation. British Medical Journal (2 Sept): 62

Milunski A 1988 First trimester screening for chromosome defects. American Journal of Obstetrics and Gynecology 159(5): 1209–1213

Pearce J 1987 Ultrasound in early pregnancy. Practitioner 231: 85–92

Quinlan R W, Cruz A C, Martin M 1983 Hydramnios: ultrasound diagnosis and its impact on perinatal management and pregnancy outcome. American Journal of Obstetrics and Gynecology 145(3): 306–311

Raphael D D 1988 Handicapped infants: medical ethics and the law. Journal of Medical Ethics 14(1): 5–10

Scholtz C et al 1990 Decision for and against the utilisation of amniocentesis and chorion villus biopsy. Journal of Psychology, Obstetrics and Gynaecology (suppl) (Dec): 27–40

Spagnola A 1990 Identity and status of the human embryo. Ethics and Medicine 6(3): 42

Ward R H, Modell B, Petrou M, Karagözlu F, Douratsos E 1983 Method of sampling chorionic villi in first trimester of pregnancy under guidance of real time ultrasound. British Medical Journal 286: 1542–1544

Wiever J et al 1990 Audit of amniocentesis from a district hospital: is it worth it? British Medical Journal 300: 1243–1245

15 The fetal skull

Unlike most other bones, the bones comprising the vault of the fetal skull are formed from membrane and not from cartilage. In this membrane are five points called **ossification centres** (Fig. 15.1A).

The first signs of early skull development occur at the end of the 4th week of intrauterine life and commence in the occiput. As pregnancy advances, calcium is laid down around these centres and so the skull bones begin to develop. Calcification begins as early as the 5th week following conception (Fig. 15.1B).

The chief function of the skull is to protect the brain which lies within it and when the skull bones have completely ossified, the bones of the vault are much more dense than those of the face.

When a premature infant is born, the bones are still far from being completely ossified and the head is said to feel rather like a table tennis ball because it can be indented. Intracranial damage is much more likely to be sustained during premature delivery because of the soft bones and the wide gaps of membrane still left not ossified (Fig. 15.1C).

At full term there are still narrow areas of membrane between the bones where ossification is still incomplete. The bones are harder than those of the premature infant and this head is compared with the hardness of a tennis ball. Incomplete ossification is advanta-

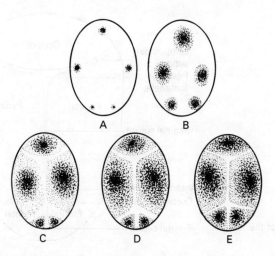

Fig. 15.1 Development of fetal skull – progressive.

geous because it allows the skull bones to overlap slightly when the head is compressed and pushed through the pelvis by uterine contractions (Fig. 15.1D).

Further ossification occurs if the fetus remains in the uterus for longer than 40 weeks. Consequently, not only do the bones become more dense and hard but the areas of membrane between them are very narrow indeed, so that when the head is compressed as it passes through the birth canal, the bones cannot overlap so easily, delivery is more difficult and there is an increased risk of intracranial damage (Fig. 15.1E).

The head is the leading part in about 95% of all labours and, in relation to other parts of the fetus, it is not only the largest, but the most resistant part.

For descriptive purposes, the fetal skull is divided into three regions:

The vault (Fig. 15.2)

The area above an imaginary line drawn from below the occipital protuberance to the orbital ridges. A knowledge of its features is very necessary in the practice of obstetrics, as this chapter will show.

The face The area extending from the orbital ridges to the junction of the chin and neck. It is composed of 14 bones which are firmly united.

The base The bones in this area are also firmly united and help to protect the brain.

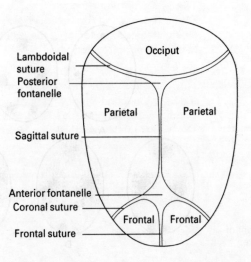

Fig. 15.2 Vault of the fetal skull.

Lambdoidal suture
Posterior fontanelle
Occiput
Parietal
Parietal
Sagittal suture
Anterior fontanelle
Coronal suture
Frontal
Frontal
Frontal suture

Bones

The occiput
One bone which lies posteriorly. The ossification centre can be easily defined and is named the **occipital protuberance**.

The parietals
Laterally, on the right and left are the parietal bones with their ossification centres, the **parietal eminences**.

The frontals
Anteriorly lie the right and left frontal bones, whose ossification centres are named **frontal eminences** or **frontal bosses**.

Sutures

A suture is an area of membrane between the skull bones where ossification has not been completed.

Lambdoidal suture:
lies between the occiput and the parietal bones.

Sagittal suture
divides the parietal bones.

Coronal suture
separates the parietal bones from the frontal bones.

Frontal suture
divides the frontal bones.

Fontanelles

These are areas where two or more sutures meet. Altogether there are six fontanelles but only two need to be mentioned here.

1. The posterior fontanelle
This occurs at the junction of the lambdoidal and sagittal sutures. It is very small and triangular in shape and does not close until the infant is 6 weeks old. On vaginal examination it can be recognised by these characteristics because it will just admit a finger tip and three sutures can be distinguished running into it. When felt on such an examination, it indicates that the fetus is lying with his chin well down on his chest and the head is therefore well flexed. This allows the smallest circumferences of the skull to pass through the birth canal.

The posterior fontanelle can be used to indicate the relationship of the fetal skull to one of the four quadrants of the mother's pelvis (i.e. right and left anterior and right and left posterior quadrants.) Thus if the posterior fontanelle is felt on the right-hand side of the mother's pelvis and towards the front, the occiput must be lying in the right anterior quadrant of the pelvis and the fetal position is said to be right occipitoanterior

2. The anterior fontanelle
This is formed where the sagittal, coronal and frontal sutures meet and it is diamond-shaped. It is much larger than the posterior fontanelle, being approximately 2.5 cm in length and 1.3 cm wide. The shape and size therefore help to identify it on vaginal examination, as does the palpation of four suture lines. When this fontanelle is felt on such an examination it proves that the fetal head is not well flexed and a larger circumference is attempting to pass through the birth canal. Labour on this occasion is likely to be prolonged and more difficult. The anterior fontanelle should be completely ossified by the time that the infant is 18 months of age.

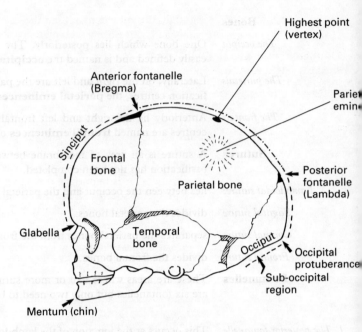

Fig. 15.3 Area of the fetal skull.

| **Areas of the skull** (Fig. 15.3) | *Glabella*: the bridge of the nose. |

Glabella: the bridge of the nose.
Sinciput: the forehead.
Bregma: the anterior fontanelle.
Vertex: the highest point on the fetal skull. It lies on the sagittal suture midway between the parietal eminences. The term vertex is also used to describe an area bounded by the anterior and posterior fontanelles and the parietal eminences.
Lambda: the posterior fontanelle.
Occiput: the area occupied by that bone.
Suboccipital area: lies below the occipital protuberance.
Mentum: the chin.

Circumferences of the fetal skull

A well-flexed head
When the fetus lies with his head well flexed, the circumference which attempts to pass through the pelvis, i.e. to engage in the pelvis, is the suboccipitobregmatic circumference of 30 cm. The measurement is taken around the occipital protuberance, the parietal eminences and the bregma. It is a circular area and passes through the pelvis easily.

An erect head
The circumference which engages in the pelvis is the occipitofrontal circumference of 33 cm. It is measured around the posterior fontanelle, parietal eminences, and the orbital ridge. This is not a circular area but much more ovoid, and labour is more difficult born because of the larger measurement and the shape.

A partly extended head
The circumference which tries to engage in the pelvis is the mentovertical. It measures 38 cm and is therefore too large to pass

through. It is measured around the chin and up to the vertex and is associated with a brow presentation.

Diameters of the fetal skull (Fig. 15.4A, B)

1. Biparietal   Taken between the parietal eminences and measures 9.5 cm. It is the widest transverse diameter and the fetal head is said to be engaged when the biparietal diameter has passed through the pelvic brim. In the second stage of labour, 'crowning' of the head is said to have occurred when the wide biparietal diameter of the fetal skull distends the perineum and the fetal head no longer recedes between contractions. It is important then, to maintain flexion of the head, so that the suboccipitobregmatic diameter of 9.5 cm distends the perineum and the head is slowly extended as the larger suboccipitofrontal diameter is freed.

2. Bitemporal   is measured between the two extreme points of the coronal suture and is 8 cm.

3. Suboccipitobregmatic   is the measurement from below the occiput to the bregma. It measures 9.5 cm and is associated with a normal presentation and position of the fetus, the head being well flexed.

4. Suboccipitofrontal   The head is less well flexed and the measurement of 10 cm is taken between the suboccipital region and the centre of the sinciput. This

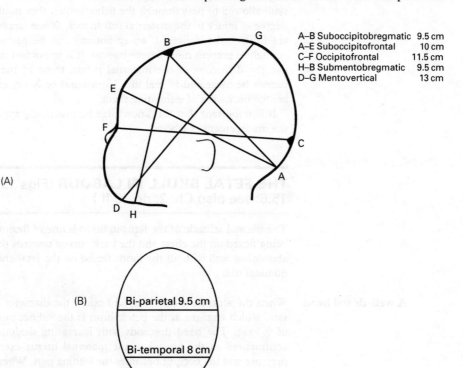

A–B Suboccipitobregmatic	9.5 cm
A–E Suboccipitofrontal	10 cm
C–F Occipitofrontal	11.5 cm
H–B Submentobregmatic	9.5 cm
D–G Mentovertical	13 cm

(A)

(B)   Bi-parietal 9.5 cm

Bi-temporal 8 cm

Fig. 15.4A and B Diameters of the fetal skull.

head will flex with good uterine contractions and labour is likely to be normal.

5. Occipitofrontal   The head is erect. The diameter attempting to engage in the pelvis is 11.5 cm, measured between the occiput and the glabella. As well as the larger diameter, the ovoid shape makes it more difficult to get through the pelvis and when the head is in this attitude labour tends to be prolonged.

6. Mentovertical   The head is partly extended, with the brow presenting. The engaging diameter is measured from the chin to the vertex and, being 13 cm, is the largest diameter of the fetal skull. Vaginal delivery when the fetal head is in this attitude is usually impossible.

7. Submentobregmatic   The head is fully extended and, as it is thrown right back, it is the face which attempts to pass through the pelvis. The measurement of 9.5 cm is taken from below the chin to the bregma. Although this is a small diameter, labour is usually more difficult because the face bones are firmly united and cannot override; also the irregular features of the face cannot be applied well to the cervix and cannot therefore stimulate good uterine contractions.

Sutures and fontanelles recognised on vaginal examination will denote whether the head is well flexed, not flexed, or extended. The diameter of the head likely to pass through the pelvis can be calculated and, at delivery, the smallest possible diameter of the skull allowed to pass through the pelvic outlet, thus minimising the degree of injury to the maternal soft tissues. When larger diameters are likely to be delivered, an episiotomy can be performed early enough to prevent more severe trauma. It is important to note that, like the diameters of the maternal pelvis, those of the fetal skull cannot be measured in real life. Ultrasound or X-ray examination are the only ways of estimating them.

It is important that this knowledge be practically applied during the management of labour.

THE FETAL SKULL IN LABOUR (Figs 15.5 and 15.6; see also Ch. 2, pp 38 ff.)

The normal attitude of the fetus in utero is one of flexion, the head being flexed on the chest and the back curved towards the maternal abdominal wall with all the limbs flexed on the fetal chest and abdominal wall.

A well-flexed head   When the attitude is one of good flexion, the diameter of the fetal skull which engages in the pelvic brim is the suboccipitobregmatic of 9.5 cm. The head descends with increasing flexion as uterine contractions in the fundus of the maternal uterus exert fetal axis pressure and the occiput becomes the leading part. When it reaches the pelvic floor, the occiput rotates to the front and so lies beneath the pubic arch.

In the second stage of labour 'crowning' of the head occurs when its biparietal diameter distends the perineum and the head no longer recedes between contractions.

An erect head or military attitude

When the head is in the erect attitude, the engaging diameter is the occipitofrontal, 11.5 cm. It is more frequently associated with the occipitoposterior position. The possible outcome of labour is as follows:

1. Descent with increasing flexion

In about 90% of these labours the erect head descends through the pelvis with increasing flexion so that the suboccipitobregmatic diameter presents by the time the head reaches the pelvic floor and the occiput becomes the leading part. The occiput undergoes long rotation when it reaches the pelvic floor and comes to lie under the pubic arch and delivers as an occipitoanterior position.

2. Descent with no flexion of the head

A failure of the head to flex as it descends through the pelvis results in the occipitofrontal diameter (11.5 cm) being arrested in the transverse diameter of the pelvic outlet (11 cm). Rotation and descent of the head then becomes impossible as it is obstructed by the ischial spines. Manual rotation of the head or Kielland's forceps rotation with forceps delivery is then the most likely outcome.

3. Descent of head with incomplete flexion

Labour commences (as with the first two examples) with the occipitofrontal diameter of the head engaged in the pelvic brim. In this instance, however, fetal axis pressure results in the sinciput becoming the leading part. On reaching the pelvic floor the sinciput rotates anteriorly and comes to lie under the pubic arch while the occiput rotates into the hollow of the sacrum. With this type of mechanism the measurements of the fetal skull are usually relatively favourable in comparison with the size of the mother's pelvis and spontaneous delivery occurs – but with a difference!

Because the fetal head is not flexed, the long occipitofrontal diameter, together with the wide biparietal diameter, distends the perineum; the hard occiput, because it is lying posteriorly, also causes considerable pressure, and there is an excessive dilatation of the anus. The midwife with a practical working knowledge of these facts will recognise that bruising and excessive stretching of perineal tissues is inevitable, and will suggest to the mother, in good time, that an episiotomy is advisable.

Delivery is managed by allowing the smallest possible diameters of the head to distend the perineum. Once the sinciput appears under the pubic arch then flexion of the head is maintained until the vertex and then the occiput can be slowly released over the perineum. Only then is the head allowed to extend and the nose, mouth and chin are released from under the pubic arch. This condition is described as **unreduced occipitoposterior position** or **face to pubes**.

4. Descent with slight extension – brow presentation

When the head is partly extended, the engaging diameter is the mentovertical (13 cm) and the presentation is the brow. The maternal pelvis cannot accommodate this large diameter and delivery is effected by caesarean section, otherwise labour becomes obstructed. In a few instances, uterine contractions result in full extension of the head and then vaginal delivery, as face presentation is possible providing the chin lies anteriorly.

5. Descent with full extension – face presentation

Uterine contractions result in full extension of the head, converting the engaging occipitofrontal diameter to the smaller submentobregmatic (9.5cm). The chin then becomes the leading part. Providing that the chin descends to the pelvic floor and rotates anteriorly, spontaneous vaginal delivery occurs as a face presentation.

Recognising this, during delivery, the midwife maintains pressure on the sinciput until the chin is free so that the submentovertical diameter (11.5 cm), instead of the larger mentovertical diameter, distends the soft tissues. But it is inevitable that the wide transverse biparietal diameter (9.5 cm) and the hard occiput will distend the perineal tissues and an elective episiotomy should be performed to minimise the trauma.

Aftercoming head of the breech presentation

Where caesarean section or forceps delivery to the aftercoming head is not the method of delivery, it is important that, once the infant's trunk has been delivered, he is allowed to hang by his own weight for 1–2 minutes. The midwife should not exert any traction on the trunk at this time.

Various delivery manoeuvres are described in midwifery textbooks, but the object of them all is to bring the infant's head through the maternal pelvis in an attitude of flexion until his hair line is visible. Allowing the infant's trunk to hang unsupported utilises the weight of his own body to exert adequate, but minimal, traction to achieve this objective. Once his head is in the pelvic cavity, his body falls slightly and the nape of the neck appears under the symphysis pubis. The suboccipital region of the skull now occupies the area under the pubic arch. The infant's feet are now grasped by the midwife and his body is swung over the mother's abdomen so that his head is delivered following the direction of the curve of the birth canal. Slow, controlled delivery of the head is now essential. As the body is taken up through an arc of 180°, the infant's mouth, nose and then sinciput are delivered. This is a skilled manoeuvre and, if it is not carried out correctly, the consequences can be grievous:

1. Too great a degree of traction (if the midwife pulls on the infant's trunk) can cause **extension of the infant's head** as it comes through the pelvic brim.

2. Too great a 'tug' on the cervical vertebrae or allowing them (instead of the suboccipital region) to pivot under the pubic arch can result in **cervical dislocation or fracture** and **crushing of the spinal cord**.

3. **Intracranial haemorrhage** can result from the rapid compression and decompression of the head if delivery is not slow and controlled, because moulding is rapid and takes place in an upwards direction. The slow moulding which takes place during

labour over a matter of hours with a cephalic presentation is impossible when the breech presents. Yet, on the other hand, the head must be delivered as soon as possible after the body or the infant will suffer asphyxia.

4. **Asphyxia** may be a consequence of umbilical cord compression as the head enters the pelvis or due to premature inspiration of mucus or liquor before the mouth or nose are freed.

It is important to note that the exact diameters of the fetal skull cannot be measured except by radiography or ultrasound but a knowledge of their measurements is essential for the practical management of labour.

The cerebral membranes and venous sinuses (Fig. 15.5) The cerebral membranes are composed of dura mater, which is the outer of the three meninges covering the brain and spinal cord. It is a tough fibrous membrane which dips down between the brain substance and separates the cerebral hemispheres (Fig. 15.5).

The falx cerebri This is a double fold of dura mater which dips down between the two portions of the cerebrum, the largest part of the brain. The lower edge of the falx hangs loose – it is unattached.

The tentorium cerebelli This is a fold of dura mater which runs horizontally at right angles to the falx cerebri, with which it unites. Being shaped rather like a horseshoe it divides the cerebrum from the cerebellum.

The superior longitudinal sinus This is a vessel which runs posteriorly along the convex border of the falx cerebri, increasing in size as it approaches the occipital protuberance. It receives the superior cerebral veins and veins from the pericranium.

The inferior longitudinal sinus A vessel contained within the free border of the falx cerebri which also increases in size as it runs posteriorly. It receives veins from the falx and there is some drainage into it from the medial aspects of the brain.

The straight sinus This is a continuation of the inferior longitudinal sinus and lies at the junction of the falx and tentorium. It drains not only the inferior longitudinal sinus but also the great vein of Galen.

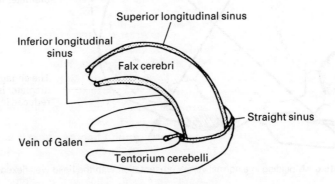

Fig. 15.5 Cerebral membranes and blood vessels.

The vein of Galen   This joins the straight sinus at its junction with the inferior longitudinal sinus and is made up of many vessels from the brain substance. If cerebral membranes are torn in the region of their junction, the vein may well be ruptured and intracranial haemorrhage may ensue.

During labour, when the fetal head must adapt itself to the shape of the birth canal, these structures are all subject to some degree of pressure as the head changes shape, but normally they are able to withstand the stress of a normal vaginal delivery.

Moulding   This is the term used to describe the change which takes place in
(Figs 15.6 and 15.7)   the shape of the fetal skull as it passes through the birth canal. Every baby's head is therefore moulded to some extent unless he is delivered by elective caesarean section. As the head descends through the pelvis in response to the downward pressure of uterine contractions, so the skull bones overlap each other. The engaging diameter of the head receives the pressure and is therefore reduced in size, while the diameter which lies at right angles to it is pushed outwards to become elongated. The shape of the baby's head following delivery is characteristic of the attitude of the head at the beginning of labour. Providing that moulding takes place gradually without being prolonged, the cerebral membranes and blood vessels are not likely to be damaged.

In certain types of moulding, however, the internal structures are more likely to be damaged. Oedema and congestion may give rise to signs of mild cerebral irritation, while tearing of the membranes with involvement of blood vessels will cause more severe signs and can lead to death or permanent cerebral damage. The dangerous types of moulding are:

1. Excessive moulding   This will occur when labour is prolonged, due to disproportion between the size of the fetal head and the maternal pelvis, or where

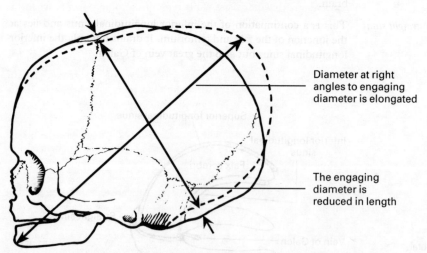

Diameter at right
angles to engaging
diameter is elongated

The engaging
diameter is
reduced in length

Fig. 15.6   Moulding in a normal vertex presentation with the head well flexed.

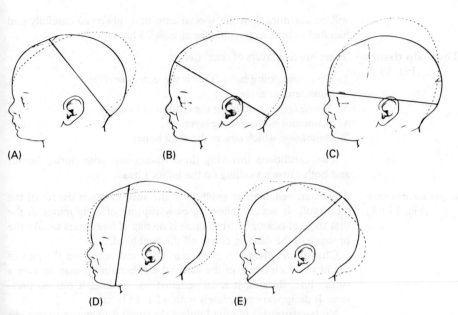

Fig. 15.7 Moulding of the fetal skull: (A) well-flexed head (B) partially flexed head (C) deflexed head (D) face presentation (E) brow presentation.

the skull bones are not completely ossified (as in prematurity) and therefore offer little resistance to pressure.

2. Upward moulding When the occipitofrontal diameter is the engaging diameter, moulding occurs in the submentobregmatic direction, so that the falx cerebri is pulled upwards. It is then likely to tear at its junction with the tentorium, and rupture of the membranes in this area will also involve the large blood vessels, resulting in intracranial haemorrhage. This type of moulding occurs when the baby delivers in the persistent occipitoposterior position and when the aftercoming head of the breech passes through the pelvis.

3. Rapid moulding Rapid compression and decompression of the head is the commonest cause of rupture of the cerebral membranes. Rapid moulding occurs in a precipitate delivery, i.e. when labour occurs within 4 hours, and during the delivery of the head of a breech presentation, because the head passes through the pelvis in a matter of minutes. It is not the tearing of the membrane which is important but the haemorrhage which occurs if the blood vessels are involved.

Any infant who has been subject to severe moulding will suffer some degree of asphyxia at birth as a result of intracranial compression. Any such infant, or one who shows signs of cerebral irritation, should be seen immediately by a paediatrician, who will most likely prescribe i.m.i. vitamin K (phytomenadione) 0.5–1 mg depending upon the infant's weight and condition. The infant will be cot-nursed in the special care unit, observed carefully and handled as little as possible for at least 24 hours.

The scalp tissues
(Fig. 15.8)

There are five layers of scalp tissue:

1. *Skin*: containing hairs. This is the outer covering
2. *Subcutaneous tissue*
3. *Muscle layer*: containing the tendon of Galea
4. *Connective tissue*: a loose layer
5. *Periosteum*: which covers the skull bones.

Two conditions involving these tissues can arise during labour and both cause a swelling on the infant's head.

Caput succedaneum
(Fig. 15.8A)

This is an oedematous swelling of the subcutaneous tissues of the fetal skull. It occurs following early rupture of membranes in the first stage of labour because there is no bag of forewaters to take the pressure of the dilating cervix off the fetal head.

Characteristics: It is present at birth and occurs on the part of the head which lies over the internal os; therefore it may lie over a suture line. Because it is an oedematous swelling, it pits on pressure. It disappears completely within 24–48 hours.

No **treatment** is required unless the caput is of excessive size but the infant should be handled as little as possible for at least 24 hours and carefully observed for signs of cerebral irritation.

Cephalhaematoma

This swelling is due to bleeding between the skull bone and the periosteum which covers it. The bleeding occurs because of friction between the skull bones and the periosteum as overriding of the bones takes place during moulding. It is just as likely to occur during a normal delivery as when a more difficult labour occurs. A low prothrombin level is probably a contributory cause.

Characteristics: It is not present at birth but appears 2–3 days afterwards, when the amount of blood is sufficient to form an obvious swelling. The swelling is limited by the periosteum and can therefore only occur over a bone, although it may be bilateral. It cannot lie over a suture. The head is usually more red and bruised in appearance than with the caput succedaneum. The swelling may increase and it takes 6 weeks at least to disappear completely.

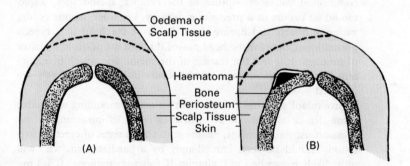

Oedema of
Scalp Tissue

Haematoma
Bone
Periosteum
Scalp Tissue
Skin

(A)   (B)

Fig. 15.8   (A) Caput succedaneum (B) Cephalohaematoma.

Treatment is only required if the haematoma increases in size over a number of days. Vitamin K injections are then given to raise the prothrombin level and assist clotting. The haemoglobin level should be estimated and the baby should be treated for anaemia if necessary.

REVISION QUESTIONS

Describe the anatomy of the fetal skull. What is moulding and why does it occur?

Write brief notes on:

1. The vertex of the fetal skull
2. Caput succedaneum
3. Cephalhaematoma.

Describe the vault of the fetal skull. How may a knowledge of its features be of value in assessing the course of labour?

How may a child's head sustain injury during spontaneous delivery? What symptoms would suggest intracranial injury, and what are the midwife's duties in such a case?

Describe the fetal skull. What changes and injuries may occur as a result of labour?

Write short notes on:

1. Engagement of the fetal head.
2. The occipitofrontal diameter of the fetal skull.
3. The increased dangers of a breech delivery.

REFERENCE AND FURTHER READING

Books

Brandt I 1989 Dynamics of head circumference growth before and after term. In: Roberts D, Thomson A (eds) Biology of fetal growth. Symposium of the Society for the Study of Human Biology, ch 15

Bibliography

GENERAL ANATOMY AND PHYSIOLOGY – BOOKS USED
THROUGHOUT
Anderson M M 1979 Anatomy and physiology of obstetrics, 6th edn. Faber
  & Faber, London
Chamberlain G 1984 Lecture notes on obstetrics, 5th edn. Blackwell
  Scientific Publications, Oxford
Garcia J et al 1985 Midwives confined. Labour ward policies and routine
  procedures. Mios conference report
Hinchcliff S M, Montague S 1988 Physiology for nursing practice. Baillière
  Tindall, London
Hudson C N 1978 The female reproductive system. Churchill Livingstone,
  Edinburgh
Llewellyn Jones D 1990 Fundamentals of obstetrics and gynaecology, 5th
  edn. Faber & Faber, London
Netter F H 1965 Reproductive system. Ciba collection of medical
  illustrations, vol 2. Ciba Foundation, New York
Polden M, Mantle J 1990 Physiotherapy in obstetrics and gynaecology.
  Butterworth-Heinemann, London
Smout C V F, Jacoby F, Lillie E W 1969 Gynaecological and obstetrical
  anatomy, 4th edn. H K Lewis, London
Wendall Smith C P, Williams P L, Treadgold S 1984 Basic human
  embryology. Pitman Medical, London
Williams P L, Warwick R, Dyson M, Bannister L H 1989 Gray's anatomy,
  37th edn. Churchill Livingstone, Edinburgh
Wilson K J W 1990 Ross & Wilson anatomy and physiology in health and
  illness, 7th edn. Churchill Livingstone, Edinburgh

Index